25 "FORBIDDEN" CURES
UNCENSORED
HEALTH
You Can Have Today

Volume 2

ALLIANCE FOR ADVANCED HEALTH

Cover Design: Robin Kean
Managing Editor: Sarah Adler

615B001138

TABLE OF CONTENTS

- Slash Your Heart Risk By Eating MORE Fried Foods?!?
- Could ONE Supplement Keep You from Ever Having a Heart Attack Again?!?
- World War II Discovery Prevents Heart Death (and the Government Was FORCED to Admit It)
- Delicious Dinner BLASTS Clogged Arteries
- 10 Foods That Stop Inflammation COLD

- Pee Like a Teenager Again with This Incredible African Bark
- Don't Let This Prostate "Gold Standard" Ruin Your Life
- The Baseball Player's Secret to Beating Prostate Cancer
- This 2-second Prostate Cancer "Test" Won't Cost You a Dime
- Underground Tips for MIND-BLOWING Sex After Prostate Surgery
- Poison Your Prostate?!? Skip This CRAZY Treatment
- 7 Superfoods That CRUSH Prostate Problems
- Forgotten Egyptian Cure ERASES Prostate Problems

- Mythical Indian Berry Gets Energy Levels Soaring
- The 7 Energy Busters Hiding in Your Medicine Cabinet
- Is a Secret Thyroid Disorder Sapping Your Energy? Take This Quiz
- Eat These 3 Superfoods for a PERFECT Thyroid
- 5 Cheap, Natural Energy Boosters You Can Start Using Today

- Is This Russian "Spy Pill" the Secret to Limitless Aging?
- Got Wrinkles? ERASE Them for 32 Cents a Day!
- Give Father Time a Run for His Money with This "Master" Antioxidant
- 90% of Women Rave About This Natural Hair-Loss Breakthrough
- The 20-Minute Secret to Living to 100 (and You Don't Have to Diet)
- Make Varicose Veins Disappear with This Old "Butcher's Remedy"
- Those Rough Fingernails Are a Canary in the Coal Mine! Here's How to Fix Them

- Get Supermodel Skin With These Oil Tricks
- STOP Vision Problems with These 5 Underground Treatments
- How to Remove Warts WITHOUT Going to the Doctor
- Hidden Natural Breakthroughs Kill Foot Fungus DEAD
- This Oil Heals Stubborn Wounds…So Why Isn't Anybody Talking About It?
- Live 20 Years Longer with This Sacred Japanese Leaf
- Give Yourself a Natural HGH Boost—Without the Needles

CHAPTER 7: 189
Erase Nagging Pain WITHOUT Drugs or Surgery

- Let This Calming Mineral Soothe Away Even the Worst Pain
- The "Devil's Secret" to Banishing Back Pain
- The Indian Chef's Trick for Smooth, Comfortable Joints
- Ease Fibromyalgia with This Baltimore Doctor's Cocktail
- Can This Odd Jewelry Stop Migraine Nausea?
- Heartbroken Dad Discovers Underground Joint Breakthrough!
- 4 Easy Home Remedies for Tension Headaches
- Is This "Vine of the Gods" the Next Rheumatoid Arthritis Breakthrough?!?
- Stop Gout Flare-Ups with This Drug-Free Protocol
- Fix Joint Woes with a Glass of "Super Water?"

CHAPTER 8: 217
Get a YOUNGER Brain with These Blacklisted Discoveries

- Can This Strange Mushroom Actually REVERSE Dementia?!?
- Did Hurricane Katrina Uncover Secret Cause of Parkinson's?!?
- Vitamin B12 For Your Brain? Throw it Out Until You Read This!
- This Superstar's Secret Could Save You from Alzheimer's
- Slow Memory Loss to a Crawl with This Vitamin Fix
- [Warning] Popular Medical Test Could Damage Your Brain
- Powerful Spice Fights Depression as Well as Prozac
- Ancient Tonic Could Keep You from Getting Parkinson's
- Weird Underwater Algae STOPS Memory Loss
- Can Eliminating This ONE Food Prevent Alzheimer's?!?
- Is Your iPhone Destroying Your Memory?
- Get a 25% Brain Boost with This Forbidden Dessert

- Chinese Breakthrough REVERSES Alzheimer's in 8 Weeks
- African Seed Fights Depression Better Than Prozac
- IGNORED Asian Cure Boosts Brain Power in 2 Hours Flat
- MEND Program Turns Back Alzheimer's in 3 Months ?!?
- Can This "Virgin Mary Secret" Restore Lost Memory?

- 7 Hay Fever Breakthroughs Big Pharma Doesn't Want You to Know About
- How to Make Your Own Cough Syrup—for Just a Couple Bucks!
- Lower Stubborn Fevers with These Folk Healers' Secrets
- Never Get the Flu (or a Flu Shot) Again
- Soothe Your Grandkids' Colds Without Dangerous Meds
- Ancient "Quack" Treatment Provides Allergy Relief
- Stop Sore Throat Pain in Just Seconds with These Proven Helpers

- Stop Bloating (and Look Thinner) in JUST ONE DAY!
- Odd (but Delicious) Soup Seals Your Leaky Gut
- Treat Your IBS Naturally with These 4 Drug-Free Breakthroughs
- Miracle Diet Soothes Even the Worst Gut Problems…So Why Haven't You Heard of It?
- Hidden Food Protein is Destroying Your Gut (and Your Health)
- The Thanksgiving Secret to Taming Ulcers

- This Natural Salt Runs Circles Around Diabetes Meds
- Lose That Sweet Tooth Forever with This Mineral Trick
- Turn Off Diabetic Nerve Pain with This Vitamin Fix
- Diabetes Breakthrough Works in 1 DAY!
- Wartime Coffee Substitute Fights Diabetes and Arthritis
- The Blood Sugar Bomb Hiding in Your Water Bottle
- Delicious (and Forbidden) Treat CRUSHES Insulin Resistance

- Skipping This Popular Bone Test Could Save Your Health
- Don't Let This "Brain Pill" Eat Your Bones Away
- This Blacklisted Treatment Could Save Your Thinning Bones
- Weird Sea Creature Unlocks Secret to TOTAL ARTHRITIS RELIEF!

- Get "Eagle Eyes" With This Powerful Supplement Combo
- Dirt-Cheap Supplement Fights Ugly Cold Sores
- Want Better Hearing? Check Your Medicine Cabinet First
- Get Control of Asthma with This Vitamin Fix
- Delicious Smoothie Fights Even the Worst Jet Lag
- The Medicine Man's Trick for Hot Flash Relief
- Take the Sting and Itch Out of Bug Bites in Just Seconds!
- 6 Natural Balms Heal Painful Sunburns
- Skip Those Miserable Detoxes—And Use This Mouthwash Instead
- Mediterranean Breakthrough Stops Hemorrhoid Pain
- This Bible King's Secret REVERSES Vision Loss

CHAPTER 1:

REVERSE CANCER WITH THESE BLACKLISTED BREAKTHROUGHS

Weird Fruit Duo is Like Kryptonite for Cancer

We all remember those old Superman comic books. Any time the Man of Steel would come into contact with kryptonite... that radioactive ore from his home planet...he'd feel his strength start to melt away.

Now picture if there were simple, natural remedies that could have the same effect on cancer cells—that could actually...

Weaken deadly cancer cells until they shrivel up and _die_!

Believe it or not, those remedies already exist. And they're being quietly used by alternative cancer doctors around the world right now.

These remarkable cancer breakthroughs are called graviola (*Annona muricata or "Muricata"*) and pawpaw (*Asimina triloba*). And they may be just the weapon that you or a loved one needs to get the upper hand in your fight against cancer.

Both graviola and pawpaw are closely related fruits that grow on trees in North and South America. And in study after study they are producing results that could turn the billion-dollar cancer industry right on its head.

Graviola and pawpaw work by starving hungry cancer cells of a vital energy source known as ATP. And you know what happens when you starve cells, right?

First they stop growing…and then they die. Fast.

Graviola, also known as soursop, is a fruit tree that grows in the Amazon regions of South America. For ages it's been used to treat infections and as a powerful antioxidant.

But now science is proving that it may be the next great cancer cure. In laboratory studies, graviola extract has been shown to attack breast, colon, lung, prostate, pancreatic, liver, and skin cancer cells. In fact, lab analysis has shown it's 3,000% more potent than chemotherapy drugs.

In other words, it attacks some of the deadliest and hard-to-treat types of cancer around.

In a 2012 study out of the University of Nebraska Medical Center, a team of scientists found that graviola kills pancreatic cancer cells dead by shutting off their metabolic fuel supply.

In fact, in a laboratory analysis, researchers could actually see the graviola going to work *in just 48 hours*! Their study proved that graviola can actually inhibit both pancreatic cancer cell growth and metastasis (or spread).

That's not just a big development…it's potentially life-saving. Pancreatic cancer is notorious for resisting conventional mainstream treatments like chemotherapy.

In fact, the 5-year survival rate for some types of pancreatic cancer is as low as 1 percent!

In another international lab study, researchers exposed prostate cancer cells to a graviola extract.

Graviola killed _nearly 100 percent_ of prostate cancer cells in just 72 hours!

That's right—nearly all cancer cells DEAD in only 3 days! And that sounds a whole lot better than conventional mainstream prostate cancer treatments like surgery or hormone therapy that can wreck your sex life or even leave you in adult diapers!

So how does graviola work for patients like you? Just ask Kathy from New South Wales, Australia. She was diagnosed with colon cancer in 2013 and says she started taking graviola a month later.

"All of my tests are clean," she writes. "Two years later, and not even a polyp was found."

And graviola's cousin pawpaw is delivering impressive results all its own.

Pawpaw is a bean-shaped fruit that grows throughout North America (it's sometimes called the "poor man's banana"). And like graviola, it practically starves cancer cells of the energy they need to survive.

One study published in 1997 found that pawpaw kills breast cancer cells that actually resist powerful mainstream drugs (but oncologists keep pushing those drugs anyway).

Scientists from the University of Mississippi discovered that, in addition to starving cancer cells' mitochondria of their energy supply, pawpaw disrupts vital pathways that these cells use to communicate and survive.

Again, this discovery was made 20 years ago—and most cancer patients have still NEVER heard about pawpaw from their doctors.

So what could pawpaw treatment mean for you? Well, here's what it did for Mary.

Mary was 70 years old and had been diagnosed with Stage IV breast cancer when she started taking daily pawpaw capsules. After just 6 weeks, she reduced her CA2729 score (a common marker for breast cancer) by an unbelievable 50 percent!

Her tumor shrank and her health was stabilized—
in a month and a half!

Even Mary's skeptical doctor was blown away by the results pawpaw delivered!

And wait until you hear about Mike, a 73-year-old man with Stage IV prostate cancer that had spread to his neck and abdomen. After the same 6 weeks on pawpaw, *Mike's tumors shrank 25 percent and his PSA levels stabilized!*

Can you just imagine the look on his doctor's face?

Both graviola and pawpaw have become critical weapons used by alternative doctors in the fight against cancer.

But because the drug companies can't make a fortune off these natural remedies (and all our government cares about is drug company profits), don't expect to see commercials for them anytime soon.

In fact, one of the recent heads of United States Food and Drug Administration, Dr. Robert Califf (appointed by President Barack Obama), previously worked as a paid researcher and consultant for Big Pharma! Some people claimed he was practically a sleeper agent!

Of course, that doesn't mean you can't start putting these natural, underground remedies to work for you.

You can buy graviola supplements from Fresh Health Nutrition at **www.freshhealthnutrition.com**

To get your hands on pawpaw, go to **www.naturessunshine.com**

This Underground Cancer Treatment Could Save Your Life

Imagine sitting with your doctor in his office…huge smiles of relief on both of your faces.

Your latest imaging results are back. And they've proven, again, that your tumor is continuing to shrink.

It's literally melting away. And you haven't had a single chemo drip or sat for any radiation sessions.

People just like you are getting these results—and they're using an alternative cancer treatment that many patients are never told about.

It's called intravenous vitamin C (IVC), and the mainstream has been trying to blacklist it for years.

Fortunately, the tide is starting to turn a bit.

You see, Nobel Prize winner Linus Pauling first proposed using vitamin C to treat cancer decades ago. That's because he understood that at high enough doses, vitamin C produces hydrogen peroxide in our bodies—and that is toxic to cancer cells.

Of course, mainstream doctors and drug companies did

everything they could to try to convince the public that Pauling was wrong…and crazy.

But we know now that he was absolutely right.

Numerous studies have now proven the cancer-killing ability of IVC, and it's used by alternative health doctors all across the country.

The University of Kansas Medical Center has developed a treatment protocol for doctors, and even the federal government has funded studies on it.

In one case, reported by federal health agencies, a 51-year-old woman with metastatic kidney cancer opted for IVC treatment. After just 7 months of twice-weekly infusions, her tumors had shrunk so dramatically that they were practically invisible on film!

In another case, a man with bladder cancer that was already spreading started getting IVC. He was completely cured—and when researchers checked in with him 9 years later, he was still in fantastic health.

What makes IVC so special as a cancer treatment is that it's incredibly versatile. In fact, a 2015 lab study out of Cornell found that it can even kill colorectal cancer cells with a genetic mutation that makes them hard to treat.

Of course, chemotherapy, surgery, and radiation are massive, multi-billion dollar industries. So many patients are never given the option of IVC.

If you want to give IVC a try, your best bet is to call alternative doctors in your market. The American College for Advancement in Medicine has a great physician locator at **www.acam.org** (look under the Resources tab).

You probably won't have to make too many calls before you find a doctor who offers it – or knows someone who does.

Make sure you ask how long the doctor has been offering

the treatment, and what his success rate has been. You always want to choose an experienced doctor you feel comfortable with.

If you're currently undergoing chemo, you should know that IVC has also been found to decrease side effects like fatigue and nausea. Any doctor can order up IVC, so talk to your doc about incorporating it into your treatment.

Indian "Garbage Weed" Destroys Liver Cancer Cells

The drug companies and mainstream medicine have spent BILLIONS trying to develop new and expensive ways to treat your cancer.

They have everything from toxic chemotherapy drugs to radiation machines designed to poison and burn the cancer right out of you.

But the next great cancer cure may be a whole lot safer—and much easier to get your hands on.

In fact, it may be growing in your backyard right now.

It's called *Solanum nigrum* or black nightshade. And it's a shrub that now grows in just about every part of the world.

And, believe it or not, it's often cut down or plucked out of the ground by people who consider it a weed or a nuisance plant.

Black nightshade is even listed as an official agricultural nuisance plant in dozens of countries around the world.

But in other parts of the world, they know better. In traditional Indian medicine, for example, black nightshade has been used for centuries to treat everything from mouth ulcers to liver problems.

And over the past several years, studies have shown that black nightshade may have a powerful ability to kill cancer cells or stop cancer from spreading.

A 2015 lab study published in the *Journal of Pharmacy and Biological Sciences* found that black nightshade extract was "cytotoxic" to cancer cells.

In other words, it was killing cancer cells DEAD and stopping them from replicating.

And in another study out of China, black nightshade slowed the growth of cervical cancer in mice.

Even more exciting, a 2016 lab study out of India compared an extract derived from black nightshade against the liver cancer drug sorafenib. The black nightshade extract was an unbelievable 10 TIMES MORE TOXIC to cancer cells.

And here's the best part—it didn't harm healthy cells at all.

Because it also has a long history of use for treating liver ailments, researchers are especially excited about black nightshade's prospects as a liver cancer treatment.

Liver cancer is one of the deadliest and hardest-to-treat cancers around. The five-year survival rate for some types of liver cancer is less than 3 percent.

If you have some black nightshade growing in your back yard, don't get too excited—it's not the kind of herb you want to mess with yourself.

Instead, look for it as an ingredient in liver care supplements (Himalaya Herbal Healthcare out of Texas at **www.himalayausa.com** is one company that uses it).

Also, look for doctors and practitioners who specialize in herbal or Ayurvedic medicine.

The American College for Advancement in Medicine (**www.acam.org**) and the National Ayurvedic Medical Association (**www.ayurvedanama.org/**) are two great places to start.

The Mammogram Secret You'll NEVER Hear From Your Doctor

Speaking out against the mammogram is a little like speaking out against Santa Claus or the Easter Bunny.

It just isn't done.

The cancer industry (and it *is* an industry) has spent a fortune promoting early detection. And if you're a woman over 40 and tell your doctor you want to skip your mammogram, he'll probably look at you like you're crazy.

But facts are facts—and there's a very ugly fact about mammograms that you'll never hear mainstream medicine admit.

A mammogram is more likely to wreck your life than save it. And countless women every year learn that the hard way.

A 2016 study out of Dartmouth found that, more often than not, mammograms are just finding small, harmless tumors that will never grow.

The tumors may be harmless—but the treatment isn't. You see, once these tumors are diagnosed, women end up with radiation, surgery and other painful and sickening treatments they don't need.

It's called "overdiagnosis," and the authors wrote that "women were considerably more likely to have tumors that were overdiagnosed."

Of course, that may seem like a risk worth taking, if a mammogram could also catch a potentially deadly cancer and save your life.

Unfortunately, there's very little evidence that mammograms are doing that at all.

A 2012 study published in the prestigious *New England Journal of Medicine* found that mammograms were detecting lots of early and non-lethal tumors, but they weren't leading to any reductions in the numbers of late-stage breast cancers.

That's the exact opposite of what you'd expect if we were catching potentially dangerous cancers early.

And a massive study out of Canada, called the Canadian National Breast Screening Study, couldn't find any evidence that mammograms were leading to any reductions in breast cancer deaths.

That's right—they poured through 25 years' worth of data and couldn't prove that mammograms were saving lives at all.

And, of course, mammograms deliver a dose of radiation that could cause cell damage and problems down the road.

If you want to continue cancer screenings, there may be safer ways to go about it. Many alternative doctors today offer digital thermography, which comes with no radiation and may do a better job of determining just how risky a tumor is.

That could save you from having your life ruined by over-treatment.

If you want to find an alternative doctor, a good place to start is the website for the American College for Advancement in Medicine at **www.acam.org**.

Are You Getting 10 TIMES MORE CHEMO Than You Need?!?

If you've ever suffered through chemotherapy treatment—or have a loved one who has—you learned an ugly truth about it really fast.

It is, quite simply, one of the most barbaric medical treatments ever invented.

You're literally trying to poison cancer cells to death. And you end up poisoning and destroying lots of other healthy cells and tissue in the process, too.

You see the effects in the mirror, as your hair falls out in clumps and you begin to waste away from constant nausea and a loss of appetite. It's a treatment that practically brings you to death's door, all to supposedly save your life.

It's no wonder that patients sometimes stop treatment completely rather than go through another round of chemo.

But what if chemotherapy didn't need to be so toxic after all? What if your doctor is actually using *10 times more chemo* than you need to treat your cancer?

Believe it or not, there's a growing army of alternative doctors who say that's the case. And they've successfully eliminated 90 percent of chemo drugs using a treatment that's actually being kept from countless cancer patients everywhere.

It's called insulin potentiation therapy (IPT) and the mainstream is doing everything it can to make sure you never hear about it.

In fact, they've been trying to silence it for nearly a century!

IPT was first invented by Dr. Donato Perez Garcia in Mexico in 1932, and it relies on a very simple and commonsense principle.

You see, insulin actually makes the membranes of diseased cancer cells more permeable. That makes it easier for medications to enter the cells and go to work.

In other words, you can get the same cancer-fighting effect while using less chemotherapy drugs.

Doctors who practice IPT say they've been able to reduce the amount of chemo drugs needed by up to 90 percent!

That means that cancer patients who are denied IPT as a treatment option are actually getting up to 10 times more chemo drugs than they need.

It's an absolute outrage. And right now, mainstream medicine is waging a war against IPT to make sure you can't get your hands on it. They're trying to discredit it at every turn, even though insulin is a perfectly legal drug for doctors to administer with cancer treatment.

The war against IPT is all about money. You see, insulin is a relatively cheap generic drug—but the mainstream makes a fortune off of chemotherapy.

In fact, just 8 weeks of chemo can cost as much as $30,000. And doctors and hospitals aren't about to accept a 90 percent hit to their margins.

Instead, they try to scare patients by claiming there isn't enough science behind IPT. But that's just nonsense.

One lab study found that insulin made chemotherapy drugs thousands of times more effective. That research was published nearly 40 years ago, and the National Cancer Institute was even involved—but it's been practically hidden away from today's cancer doctors.

A 2003 study out of China also found that insulin dramatically increased the effectiveness of chemo medications.

And in a small study on breast cancer patients, every single one of the women given IPT improved. Their tumors shrank or disappeared completely, or they were able to actually reverse the spread of their cancer.

Now, with the use of insulin, the most common risk of IPT is low blood sugar. But doctors manage that risk by injecting sugar water after treatment and monitoring patients' blood sugar.

With the kind of results IPT has produced, it should be offered as a treatment option for cancer patients everywhere. But the truth is, you'll have to do some research to locate a doctor who offers it near you.

Your best bet is to visit **www.bestanswerforcancer.org** and click the "Find a Physician" tab. Then you'll see a link to search for IPT doctors in your state.

Was This PROVEN Cancer Killer Hidden For 45 years?

Imagine a powerful compound that actually kills cancer cells on contact…that has the strength to wipe away tumors and actually reverse the progression of this deadly disease.

It may be the greatest cancer breakthrough of our lifetimes. But powerful special interests have been working for nearly half a century to make sure you can't get your hands on it.

Until now.

This powerful cancer fighter is called vitamin B17—also sometimes known as amygdalin or laetrile. And it may be the subject of one of the greatest medical cover-ups in history… one that may have left countless people to suffer or even die.

You see, B17 is a sugar compound found in the seeds of common fruits, including some that may be sitting in your refrigerator right now, like apricots, apples, and plums.

And in the early 1970s, animal research at Memorial Sloan Kettering Cancer Center in New York proved that it has the power to poison and kill potentially deadly cancer cells.

Unfortunately, that's when powerful special interests from the mainstream and the drug companies went to work.

Subsequent studies were allegedly scrapped when they started to show positive results, and serious questions were raised about Sloan Kettering's deep ties to pharmaceutical giants.

When Sloan Kettering employee Ralph Moss exposed the cover-up in 1977, he was silenced and fired. You can read about the entire scandal in his book, *Doctored Results*, available at **www.amazon.com.**

The mainstream has done everything it can to prevent cancer patients from having access to B17. But brave researchers have continued to press forward—and the results they've seen from this natural compound have been nothing short of miraculous.

A 2014 study out of Germany found that B17 was able to reduce the size and spread of bladder cancer tumors.

And two different studies looked at the effect of B17 on prostate and cervical cancer cells, and found that B17 triggered a process called cellular apoptosis.

In other words, it forced the cancer cells to commit suicide! That's because B17 seems to block some of the enzyme pathways that allow cancer cells to grow and thrive.

The team of scientists behind one of the studies claimed their research proved that B17 could be a "valuable option" for the treatment of cancer. But it's an option that thousands of cancer patients are being denied right now.

You don't need to be one of them. You can get your hands on B17 by buying apricot seeds to eat or supplements. Both are available at **www.apricotpower.com**.

If you eat the seeds, a good rule of thumb is to not eat more in one sitting than you'd get from a serving of apricot. So if you'd only eat one apricot at a time, that may be equal to 6 or 7 seeds.

Amazing Harvard Discovery *Stops* Colon Cancer?

They say that timing is everything—and when it comes to colon cancer, that's definitely the case.

When colon cancer is caught early enough, it's one of the more treatable cancers around. Catch it after it's started to spread, and the 5-year survival rate plummets.

And even if you beat colon cancer, there's a good chance you're going to spend months (or years) enduring painful and sickening treatments like chemotherapy, radiation and surgery.

As far as colon cancer is concerned, your best bet is to avoid getting it in the first place.

And Harvard scientists have discovered an incredibly easy—and completely surprising—way to do just that.

In their recent study, researchers analyzed eight years of health data for over 96,000 men and women who were in their late 60s. They were monitored for things like physical activity and supplement use.

After the researchers sorted out the data, they discovered something amazing.

Folks who took glucosamine and chondroitin, popular joint

supplements, slashed their risk of developing colon cancer by an impressive 23 percent.

That's 23 percent lower risk of developing a serious cancer that will kill 50,000 Americans this year.

And, no, your eyes aren't playing tricks on you—we're talking about the same glucosamine and chondroitin that are regularly used in joint care supplements.

Both glucosamine and chondroitin are natural substances that are found in human tissues, such as joint cartilage. And in study after study they've been found to make joints more comfortable and to even help preserve cartilage.

So how on Earth could they help fight cancer, too?

Well, glucosamine and chondroitin also help keep inflammation in check, which is one reason they work so well for joint support.

But inflammation is also a key driver for several types of cancer, including colon cancer. So by keeping your inflammation in check, you may help lower your cancer risk.

The good news about glucosamine and chondroitin is that they're often sold together, so you don't need to buy two different supplements.

Puritan's Pride makes both capsule and liquid supplements that contain both ingredients, and you can buy them at **www.puritan.com**

Glucosamine and chondroitin have both been used in natural medicine for ages, and are incredibly safe. So it's worth giving them a try—you could end up improving your joint health and slashing your cancer risk at the same time.

This "Morning Miracle" Neutralizes Oral Cancer Cells!

When you have aggressive cancer, it's a lot like having a monster growing inside your body.

And when you're dealing with oral cancer, you can literally see the monster staring back at you in the mirror every day.

Now imagine if you could literally flip an "off" switch on those mouth cancer cells...if you could sap them of their energy and even kill them off by the billions.

And imagine if you could do it without putting any of your healthy cells or tissue at risk.

Scientists say it's now possible, thanks to a powerful compound in a drink you may be enjoying every day.

It's green tea—the "morning miracle" that's been found to help prevent everything from heart disease to Alzheimer's.

Now, it looks like we can add "cancer killer" to green tea's impressive resume.

You see, green tea is packed with a powerful compound called EGCG that's already been proven to help prevent certain cancers from forming.

But now we know it can kill existing cancers, too.

For the study, published in *Molecular Nutrition and Food Research*, researchers exposed oral cancer cells to EGCG in a laboratory setting.

And the cancer cells never stood a chance!

As the cancer cells began dying off quickly, scientists realized the EGCG was attacking them in 3 different ways to practically guarantee the cancer cells couldn't survive.

For example:

1. It damaged the cells' mitochondria, which they need to produce energy to survive and grow. Think of it as hitting an "off" switch.
2. It actually created reactive oxygen species (damaging compounds) to attack the cells. It's as if it manufactured its own ammunition.
3. It took away the cancer cells' ability to fight off the damage from the reactive oxygen species. EGCG completely removed the cancer cells' natural defenses.

The end result is that the cancer cells were killed, while healthy cells weren't damaged at all.

Chemotherapy and radiation sure couldn't promise that.

With all that we've learned about the health benefits of green tea and EGCG, you'd think that every doctor in the world would be recommending them for their patients.

But, unfortunately, unless a treatment can make doctors and drug companies a fortune, the mainstream isn't interested.

Fortunately, it's really easy to put the power of green tea and EGCG to work for you. If you're not already drinking green tea, it's a good idea to start.

Drinking a couple mugs of warm green tea is one of the best things you can do for your health each day.

And you can also get EGCG concentrated as a supplement. Swanson Health Products sells EGCG supplements online at **www.swansonvitamins.com**.

Kill Cancer 3 Different Ways with This French Secret

It may be the most ironic part of becoming a senior citizen.

You reach a certain age…maybe 60, 70, or even 80…and all of the sudden, everyone starts treating you like a child!

They'll tell you what you should or shouldn't eat. They'll hound you to stop driving at night. They'll even remind you to bundle up when it's cold outside.

How do they think you made it this far in life, anyway?

And if you're like a lot of seniors, you've probably had well-meaning kids, grandkids, nieces, nephews, or even doctors who've been pestering you for years to give up alcohol.

But if you swore off red wine years ago, it's officially time to put it back on the menu. Because your favorite merlot or pinot noir is a scientifically proven health drink that could end up saving your life.

It's all because of a miraculous compound found in red grapes called resveratrol. And it's turning out to be one of the most powerful cancer fighters around.

You may have first heard about resveratrol a few decades ago, when everyone was talking about the "French Paradox."

The French love their carbs, pastries—and even cigarettes—but they still have the lowest rate of heart disease in the world.

And many health researchers believe that's because of all the heart-healthy resveratrol in all the red wine the French drink. Resveratrol is a powerful antioxidant that's been proven to prevent damage to your cardiovascular system.

But as healthy as resveratrol is for your heart, it's most impressive benefit may be as a cancer fighter.

What's *really* incredible is that this substance attacks many kinds of cancers in at least three different ways.

Dr. Colbert, a US Board Certified Physician for over 25 years, has confirmed that "Resveratrol has been proven effective in reducing the growth of breast, prostate, colon, skin, pancreatic, ovarian, liver, lung, stomach, oral, cervical, lymphatic, thyroid, as well as melanoma, leukemia, metastasis to bones."

According to a study from the American Association for Cancer Research, 70 percent of cancers are solid tumors which radiation or chemotherapy cannot penetrate. Chemo often kills a lot of tumor cells, but not all of them. Some drug-resistant cells survive...and then grow again.

The bottom line is that chemotherapy and radiation alone do not always stop the progression of the disease. Not to mention the fact that chemo also affects healthy cells, leading to horrible side effects.

So what if there was an alternative? What if there was a way to trigger death of cancer cells without affecting healthy cells?

Well, that's where resveratrol comes in.

Unlike chemotherapy drugs, it isn't toxic to healthy cells. And it doesn't fight cancer through just one mechanism. It triggers cancer death through three cellular mechanisms. As a result, cancer cells find it harder to resist resveratrol.

Cancer Killing Mechanism #1: Resveratrol Stimulates Death of Cancer Cells

Did you know your body already has a cancer fighting mechanism?

They're called natural killing (NK) cells, and they're part of our immune system. As our first line of defense against cancer cells, they bind to cancer cells, then deliver a lethal dose of toxins that trigger apoptosis (programmed cell death), killing cancer on contact.

Cancer patients usually have impaired NK cells, and for that reason, cancer cells divide and grow uncontrollably.

That's where resveratrol packs a powerful punch.

It has been demonstrated that resveratrol activates natural killing cells and increases their toxicity against cancer cells. Imagine putting NK cells on steroids and turning your own body into a cancer killing machine...that's what resveratrol does.

Cancer Killing Mechanism #2: Resveratrol Cuts Blood Supply To Tumor Cells, Starving Them To Death

Cancer cells are hungry little things, and they fuel their rapid growth by increasing the consumption of their favorite food, glucose. They also develop new blood vessels that facilitate the delivery of sugars and other nutrients to the tumor site. That's how cancer cells are able to grow uncontrollably.

But what if we could cut the supply of nutrients to the tumor site?

It turns out that's another way resveratrol fights cancer. It inhibits the growth of new blood vessels, starving cancer cells to death. Without fuel, tumors shrink...and eventually vanish.

Cancer Killing Mechanism #3: Resveratrol Turns off Enzymes That Cause Inflammation

Chronic inflammation is associated with up to 25 percent of all cancers. Scientists all agree that an enzyme called COX-2 causes inflammation, and that inflammation is a cancer promoting event. In other words, COX-2 has been linked to cancer.

Now, if there was a way to turn off the COX-2, it would attack the real root of cancer...not just its symptoms. That's exactly what resveratrol does.

Research from Memorial Sloan-Kettering showed that resveratrol completely turned off the COX-2 driver.

Andrew Dannenberg and his colleagues from New York Presbyterian Hospital have also tested over 800 natural extracts for their ability to inhibit COX-2. They confirmed that resveratrol inhibits COX-2 activity.

As you can see, it's this three-pronged approach to fighting cancer that makes this miracle molecule so effective. It attacks cancer in ways that chemotherapy and radiation can't. It supercharges our natural killer cells, cuts blood flow to tumor sites, starving them to death, and turns off enzymes that trigger cancer-promoting inflammation.

In other words, it attacks the root cause of cancer...not the symptoms. Even better, you can also take the miracle molecule as a daily preventative.

Better still, you don't have to abandon chemo or radiation to take resveratrol. Resveratrol acts as a chemo-sensitizer (a substance that can help you overcome resistance to chemotherapy drugs) and a radiation-sensitizer (makes cancer cells more vulnerable to radiation).

Michael Nicholl, an assistant professor of surgical oncology at the University of Missouri School of Medicine, recently published studies which show that resveratrol can boost the effect of radiation treatment, "increasing the likelihood of a patient's full recovery from even the most aggressive cases of the disease."

Nicholl also stated that, "Other studies have noted that resveratrol made tumor cells more susceptible to chemotherapy and we wanted to see if it had the same effect for therapy."

Prostate tumors contain low levels of proteins that kill diseased cells. When resveratrol was introduced into the tumors, the proteins' activity increased and enabled radiation to destroy up to 97 percent of cancer cells.

Red wine is an excellent source of resveratrol, but you'll also find it in foods such as peanuts, pistachios, red and purple grapes, blueberries, cranberries, mulberries, lingonberries, and even cocoa and dark chocolate.

Of course, the best way to make sure you're getting all the resveratrol you need is through a supplement.

Innate Response makes a resveratrol supplement that you can order easily on websites like **www.iherb.com**.

This Ugly "Tree Mushroom" Wipes Out Cervical Cancer Cells

For centuries, traditional folk healers have prized many varieties of mushrooms for their medicinal qualities.

But in the mushroom world, one variety stands out from all the rest. And if you're suffering from one of the deadliest cancers around...like cervical or colon cancer...it may give you the boost you need to defeat the disease for good.

It's called the chaga mushroom, and don't expect to see it on a restaurant salad or served alongside your favorite steak. It's an ugly mushroom that grows on birch tree bark in Russia, Northern Europe, and other frigid climates.

But this is one mushroom you shouldn't judge by appearance alone. Because numerous studies have now proven that chaga mushrooms are absolutely deadly to cancer cells, and these mushrooms are now being used by alternative doctors and cancer patients all over the world.

Chaga mushrooms are loaded with vitamins and minerals, as well as antioxidants, flavonoids, polysaccharides such as beta-D glucans and other important compounds that help fight cancer.

And the research behind chaga mushrooms has been nothing short of remarkable.

Laboratory studies have proven that chaga mushroom extract can actually inhibit cancer cell growth and force cancer cells to kill themselves, especially in cases of cervical or colon cancer. And unlike mainstream treatments like chemotherapy and radiation, chaga mushrooms leave healthy cells and tissue unharmed.

Aside from all the other healthy compounds in chaga mushrooms, a big secret to their success may be a substance called betulin.

Betulin is a compound in birch bark that is believed to make the trees resistant to environmental stress. And scientists believe that the betulin absorbed by chaga mushrooms help them destroy or inhibit cancer cells.

In a 2012 study, scientists from King Saud University in Saudi Arabia and the School of Pharmaceutical Sciences in Malaysia found that betulin may actually be the next breakthrough treatment for colorectal cancers.

But, believe it or not, chaga mushrooms can help you in your fight against cancer in three more important ways by:

#1: Increasing production of white blood cells

Chaga contains beta glucans, which help the immune system by supporting the production of white blood cells. White blood cells are your body's first line of defense against diseases, including cancer. And if you or someone you love has ever suffered through chemotherapy, you know it can dangerously deplete your white blood cell count.

#2: Stopping inflammation

Inflammation can trigger the development of cancer, or make existing cancers more aggressive. Chaga is high in antioxidants and it is believed that compounds in the mushroom block the action of certain proteins that cause inflammation in the body.

#3: Shielding the body from radiation damage

Chaga mushrooms can actually help reduce some of the damage your healthy cells and tissue suffer from radiation treatment. Animal studies have shown that chaga can lessen radiation side effects and even extend survival time.

So how do you get your hands on this miracle chaga mushroom?

You can get dried chaga or even chaga powder from Oregon Mushrooms Corp. at **www.oregonmushrooms.com**

One of the easiest ways to enjoy chaga is as a tea. To make the tea, heat 8-10 cups of water up slowly to 120F degrees and add 5 golf ball chunks of chaga mushrooms to it.

Let sit on a low temperature for 6 hours or longer, and drink 3 cups a day.

Fighting Cancer?
Add These 7 Foods to Your Diet

When you're fighting cancer, you'll get an earful about all the mainstream treatments available. But eating the right foods can make a huge difference and can give your body the tools it needs to beat the disease.

Here are 7 foods you can incorporate into your diet that have been proven to help fight cancer.

Cancer-Fighting Food #1: Garlic

Garlic is becoming known as a superfood due to its ability to help the body in so many ways. It boosts the immune system, helps with digestion, contains natural antibiotics and can help prevent cancer. Garlic is particularly good as a cancer preventative in the digestive system.

Cancer-Fighting Food #2: Broccoli

Another wonderful food with many health benefits is broccoli, which, along with other cruciferous vegetables, contain cancer-fighting abilities. Broccoli also contains high levels of a compound called sulforaphane, which can help the body get rid of harmful chemicals and boost immune properties. Broccoli is one of those foods that you really can't eat too much of, so load up.

Cancer-Fighting Food #3: Berries

Berries are not only loaded with immune boosting vitamin C, but also with antioxidants that are known to stop the creation of free radicals in the body that can promote cancer. As a general rule with berries, the darker the better (and healthier).

Cancer-Fighting Food #4: Tomatoes

Another great source of fiber and vitamin C, tomatoes also contain one of the highest concentrations of lycopene in any food. Lycopene is a carotenoid that, besides making tomatoes red, can stop endometrial cancer growth and help prevent cancers in the prostate and stomach. Unlike most vegetables that are best eaten raw, cooking actually increases the concentration of lycopene. Just avoid canned tomatoes.

Cancer-Fighting Food #5: Green tea

The more we learn about green tea, the better it gets. On top of all the other known health benefits of green tea, it contains a particular antioxidant that can help prevent cancer. Black tea also contains these antioxidants (known as catechins), but there is a much higher concentration in green tea.

Cancer-Fighting Food #6: Walnuts

Not the most popular nut in the pantry, walnuts can be one of the healthiest. Walnuts contain phytosterols that can block estrogen receptors in the cells of breast cancers. These molecules can slow cancer cell growth in breasts and prostates. Try to grab a handful of walnuts a day.

Cancer-Fighting Food #7: Whole grains

Whole-grain foods such as whole-grain bread, oatmeal, and brown rice contain fiber and antioxidants that can lower your risk of cancer. While you don't want to overload the body with too many carbohydrates, you should supplement every meal with a serving of whole grains.

Underground Enzyme Treatment SHUTS OFF Cancer Cells

It's Been Ignored For More Than 100 Years...But You Can Get Your Hands On It NOW!

If you or someone you love is suffering from cancer, you know that mainstream medicine only offers three options.

Cut, poison, or burn.

They'll cut out the tumors with **painful, disfiguring surgeries**...poison cancer cells (and healthy tissues) with **sickening chemotherapy**...or try to burn them with **scorching radiation**. And lots of times, after all this suffering, the cancer comes back anyway!

But more than 100 years ago, a brilliant European physician named Dr. John Beard tried to change all of that.

In 1906 he figured out that a special type of gut enzymes... known as **proteolytic enzymes**...could seek out and destroy cancer cells.

In fact, they can practically flip an "off switch" that **shuts off cancer and keeps it from spreading.**

There should be hospitals named after Dr. Beard. But instead he was shunned...and even called crazy.

Mainstream medicine continues to deny his work, and proteolytic enzyme therapy (PET) has been driven practically underground.

But we know now that PET starts fighting and destroying cancer *in just weeks*.

And if you're dealing with a difficult cancer diagnosis, this is one discovery you need to know about.

Results in Just 4 Weeks!

In the 1960s, interest in alternative cancer treatments started to explode (among patients…not among the drug companies).

And one researcher, Dr. William Donald Kelley, picked up where Dr. Beard had left off.

Dr. Kelley actually used PET to **cure** *his own cancer*.

And, from there, he began using PET to treat other patients. In fact, Kelley claims to have treated more than 33,000 patients with a **93 percent success rate!**

What's more? He saw these results in as little as 4 to 6 weeks.

Despite his incredible success, like Beard before him, Kelley was largely ignored by the mainstream medical community.

But then PET got a major boost—from the Ivy League of all places!

Starting in 1981 Dr. Nicholas J. Gonzalez of Cornell University Medical College started taking a second look at Kelley's work.

Gonzalez performed an analysis of 50 of Kelley's patients who had initially been diagnosed with 26 types of poor prognosis cancers.

These were people who mainstream medicine practically left for dead!

Thanks to PET, **all 50 patients** reversed their disease and had enjoyed long-term survival.

Again, this is just a fraction of the people who were helped by Kelley and PET.

The results were so impressive that in 1993, Gonzalez was invited to share his findings with the Cancer Therapy Evaluation Program at the National Cancer Institute (NCI). He even got some funding for his research.

But that was 25 years ago. And mainstream medicine still REFUSES to accept PET as a cancer treatment.

In fact, you have a better chance of finding gold in your backyard than locating a mainstream doctor who uses PET… or even knows about it.

Word has traveled slowly. And you can bet that the drug companies that make a fortune off of chemotherapy medicines have had something to do with that.

But once you understand how PET works…and the simple science behind it…you'll be rushing to try it for yourself.

How to Modify Your Diet to Boost PET

There are changes you can make to your diet to make PET more effective.

But those changes depend on the type of cancer you have.

From his research, Dr. Nicholas J. Gonzalez found that different cancers react differently to each dietary path.

A plant-based diet is beneficial for someone with epithelial tumors like lung, pancreas, colon, prostate, and uterine cancers. These patients are prescribed a largely vegetarian diet with minimal to no animal protein.

A meat-based diet, on the other hand, is more effective for someone with blood or immune based tumors like leukemia, myeloma, or lymphoma. These patients benefit from a high-animal protein, high-fat diet with minimal-to-moderate plant foods.

Help Your Body DESTROY Cancer Cells

The best way to beat cancer isn't to flood your body with poisons like chemotherapy.

You want to help your body find and destroy cancer cells naturally.

That's where enzymes...like the kind used in PET...come into the picture.

Enzymes are crucial to supporting your immune system and fighting diseases like cancer.

At any given time, there are more than 7,000 enzymatic reactions occurring within your body with the help of more than 3,000 specific enzymes.

Proteolytic enzymes are important to digestive health...but they do a lot more than that.

They help control inflammation in your body, which is a major contributor to cancer and other diseases.

And that's not all.

You see, cancer cells have a thick outer coating called fibrin.

Fibrin is what keeps your immune system from finding and killing these cancer cells. It also prevents chemotherapy from doing the same thing, *even at high doses*.

But proteolytic enzymes break down this fibrin so your body can identify and kill cancer cells.

And while PET is stripping away cancer cells' defenses, it is arming your body to fight them.

PET naturally boosts your immune system and increases your levels of cytokines, natural killer (NK) cells, and macrophages, which destroy unwanted invaders in your body, like cancer cells.

And here's the best part.

Malignant cancer cells actually bind to these proteolytic enzymes. This interferes with the process cancer cells need to grow and metastasize.

It's like PET shuts off cancer cells and **stops cancer dead in its tracks!**

How to Reap the Benefits of PET

There are three main types of proteolytic enzymes: pepsin, bromelain, and papain.

Pepsin occurs naturally in your gut and is essential for digestion and the breakdown of proteins.

Bromelain is found in the juice and stem of pineapple. Similar to pepsin, it is a natural digestive aid.

Papain, however, is the most important of them all and it boasts the most potent anti-cancer properties.

This type of enzyme is found in the highest concentration in the papaya fruit, especially when it is unripe.

Proteolytic enzymes can be found in other foods as well, like ginger, sauerkraut, yogurt, kefir, kiwi, and miso.

So you're probably already getting some proteolytic enzymes in your diet...just not nearly enough.

First, your body can use up these enzymes quickly through digestion and when you're fighting an illness, like cancer.

Also, once these foods are cooked or processed, the enzymes lose their effectiveness – which makes supplementing important.

PET requires regularly and aggressively supplementing with proteolytic enzymes.

If you or a loved one is struggling with a cancer diagnosis, PET may be the key to your remission and recovery.

You can find proteolytic enzymes from reputable manufacturers such as **Lucky Vitamin** and **Dr. Axe**.

The dosage, however, depends on what you are hoping to treat.

For cancer patients, experts recommend anywhere from 20 to 80 grams per day.

But for cancer prevention, only 5 to 20 grams is necessary each day.

The Area 51 Cancer Breakthrough

Buried deep in Nevada's Mojave Desert, in one of the truly remote stretches of the United States, is the most secretive military base on Earth.

The U.S. government denied its very existence for years—but today, the public knows it as Area 51.

Area 51 has been the subject of countless rumors and conspiracy theories. There's even been talk about secret alien technology being tested behind its heavily guarded perimeter.

And eventually we learned that the base is used to test highly classified military aircraft, like the U2 spy plane and the stealth bomber.

But growing throughout Area 51 may be a much larger secret…one that could set the entire cancer industry on its head.

And it's one that the federal government has kept from millions of cancer patients for decades.

It's the creosote bush, also known as chaparral. And it may be…

The greatest natural cancer killer EVER discovered.

An investigation by *Popular Mechanics* magazine reported that practically nothing is growing in the grounds of Area 51 except creosote, which survives well in the Mojave.

Just think about that…of all the land that has been cleared throughout Area 51 (and the satellite photos prove it), the government has allowed creosote to continue to flourish.

In fact, Area 51 may be the largest government-controlled supply of creosote in America. It's as if they're practically stock-piling it!

And with good reason. Because you can be certain that the U.S. government is well aware of the cancer-destroying powers of creosote.

In fact, numerous studies on its anti-cancer powers have been quietly published on the PubMed database controlled by the National Institute of Health. This is a database of medical research from around the world that most members of the American public don't know about.

And these studies are nothing short of remarkable. They prove that creosote can stop the spread of deadly cancer…and even kill cancer cells, ***starting in as little as 3 hours flat!***

Research has shown that creosote attacks cancer in three different ways:

Cancer Killing Mechanism #1: Creosote starves your cancer cells of glucose. You see, sugar is like rocket fuel for cancer cells…and without it, they can't live. By keeping cancer cells from using glucose, creosote makes sure they die by the millions…and FAST.

Cancer Killing Mechanism #2: Creosote blocks key receptors that cancer cells depend on to grow and reproduce. It's especially effective at blocking these receptors for breast and prostate cancers.

Cancer Killing Mechanism #3: Creosote actually yanks apart cancer cell DNA, keeping the cells from replicating and forcing them to die.

In a 2002 lab study, researchers PROVED that a creosote extract **killed cervical and pancreatic cancer cells** in about as much time as it takes to watch a movie.

The extract began forcing cancer cells to commit suicide *in as little as 3 hours*…and by 12 hours, as many as **one-third of the cancer cells were dying!**

If someone you love has ever had pancreatic or cervical cancer, you know that they're absolute killers.

The survival rate for some types of pancreatic cancer is a measly 1%…and **an American woman dies of cervical cancer *every 2 hours.***

And creosote has also shown powerful results against breast cancer.

A quarter-million women are diagnosed with breast cancer each year…including wives, mothers, sisters, daughters, and friends that we all know.

One out of every 8 women will be diagnosed with invasive breast cancer at some point in her life…it's practically an epidemic.

But all the way back in 2002, our government had access to a lab study from the Northwestern University Medical School… one of the top medical schools in America…that **PROVES a creosote extract kills breast cancer cells.**

The authors wrote that the extract "induced apoptosis" on breast cancer cell lines.

That means it **forced breast cancer cells to commit suicide**…and our government has had this information for 15 years!

And a 2005 study conducted by California researchers proved that creosote extract can **stop aggressive breast cancer cells from spreading!**

It actually blocks something called RTKs, which are receptors cancer cells need to survive and reproduce.

And this is just the tip of the iceberg. Researchers have

shown that creosote can help fight **lung cancer, prostate cancer, skin cancer**…and more!

The secret to creosote appears to be a compound found in the plant known as nordihydroguaiaretic acid (NDGA). It's become the subject of a great deal of research in recent years, and scientists believe it also may hold promise for treating heart disease and neurological disorders.

You can harness the power of NDGA and the amazing chaparral bush by purchasing Chaparral Liquid Extract from Hawaii Pharm at **www.hawaiipharm.com**.

"Miracle of the Magi" Wipes Out Cancer Cells in 24 Hours

Imagine a world where you and your loved ones never need to worry about cancer again...one where this dreaded disease can be destroyed with something so simple (and safe) that more than a billion people cook with it.

It all may be possible, thanks to one of the most memorable—and, researchers believe, misunderstood—passages from the Holy Bible.

You've undoubtedly read the story of the birth of Jesus countless times, and about the gifts his family received. In Matthew 2:11 it states:

"On coming to the house, they saw the child with his mother Mary, and they bowed down and worshipped him. Then they opened their treasures and presented him with gifts of gold, frankincense and myrrh."

But now Christian researchers believe that this age-old verse may have been misinterpreted...and, in fact, it may hold the key to...

A medical breakthrough that DESTROYS cancer cells in as little as 24 hours flat!

You see, the gift of "gold" may not have been gold at all, but a golden-colored spice (much more keeping with the times) known as turmeric. You see, in biblical times, people called turmeric GOLD—due to its GOLDEN color.

Turmeric is a favorite spice in Indian cuisine, and you may even have some in your cupboard right now. But turmeric, and its active ingredient curcumin, can do a lot more than add kick to your favorite dish.

In fact, Dr. Saraswati Sukumar, Ph.D., a medical oncologist at the prestigious Johns' Hopkins University School of Medicine, says, "We have close to 300 publications that cite [turmeric] for its anti-cancer effects."

And how well does this golden spice work for real people like you? Just ask 78-year-old grandfather Allan T. from Sarasota, Florida.

Doctors told Allan that his colon cancer was "incurable." He was sent home to die.

In desperation, he turned to turmeric, the "Miracle of the Magi."

Less than four months later, a hospital scan revealed Allan's cancer had vanished.

His tumors were gone…like they never even existed in the first place.

Over the moon, he gushed, "There is no question in my mind that [it] saved my life."

And that's not all. According to a study published in the *British Journal of Cancer*, a turmeric extract made esophageal cancer cells in a lab "digest themselves" within 24 hours!

In fact, leading clinics all over the place are already

prescribing it as treatment. Places like:

- The Advanced Rejuvenation Institute in Atlanta
- Westcoast Integrative Health in North Vancouver, Canada
- The Cancer Center for Healing in Irvine, California

There are more than 5,600 studies reviewing turmeric's laundry list of health properties.

In fact, research confirms the "Miracle of the Magi" contains at least:

- 20 antibiotic compounds
- 14 cancer preventatives
- 12 anti-tumor compounds
- 12 anti-inflammatory compounds
- 10 antioxidant compounds

And now, some 2,000 years later, we're only just starting to unlock turmeric's full healing potential.

Regarding its anti-cancer effects, Bharat Aggarwal, Ph.D., at the University of Texas says, "We have not been able to find a cancer we can't effectively treat in the laboratory."

Dr. Joseph Maroon, M.D., a neurosurgeon at the #1 ranked hospital in Pittsburgh, adds, "It's similar to drugs, but with none of the side effects of drugs."

The secret to turmeric, and the curcumin it contains, is that it blocks inflammation, the key driver of many chronic diseases—including cancer.

By blocking the main culprit of inflammatory response (something called "molecule NF-kappaB"), it shrinks cancer-causing inflammation.

The journal Oncogene reports it's as effective as at least 10 anti-inflammatory drugs.

So how can you start getting your hands on this "Miracle of the Magi?" Well, adding more turmeric to your diet is a great place to start.

But you can also buy supplements with a concentrated dose of curcumin, the main active compound in turmeric. You can buy TrueCurcumin highly absorbable supplements from Nature City at www.naturecity.com

Bonus Report! The Biblical Cure: Supercharge The Magi's Cancer Miracle by 2,000%.

If you want to use curcumin to help fight cancer, you want to make sure your body can absorb it as well as possible. Remember, if you don't boost absorption, you may not get a potent enough dose for the curcumin to be effective.

The first tip is to take curcumin with black pepper—that's right, just old, ordinary black pepper.

That's because black pepper contains a compound called piperine that actually enhances the absorption of curcumin. Just a quarter teaspoon of black pepper can quickly increase the bioavailability of curcumin by up to 2,000%.

There are a couple other easy ways to improve absorption of curcumin. One is to take it with fat, like whole milk or even a fish oil supplement. The fat helps curcumin to be directly absorbed into the bloodstream, bypassing the liver where much of it may be processed and unused.

Finally, you can get curcumin by eating turmeric as a root or crushed as a powder. The natural oils in turmeric also work as fats to help your body better absorb the curcumin.

CHAPTER 2:

END THE NIGHTTIME MISERY WITH THESE NATURAL SLEEP FIXES

Emperor Charlemagne's "Royal Balm" Secret to PERFECT Sleep

Especially as we get older, getting a solid eight hours of shut-eye every night can be a real challenge.

First there's the tossing and turning…and then there are the endless nighttime bathroom runs.

But if you're looking for a simple (and natural) way to get a good night's sleep, some truly effective help is on the way.

And it's all thanks to a famous emperor you probably learned about in school ages ago.

If you remember your high school history lessons, you probably know the name Charlemagne very well.

He's known as the Father of Modern Europe, and was even crowned Holy Roman Emperor in the year 800.

But what you might not know about Charlemagne is that he may be responsible for one of the greatest sleep breakthroughs ever.

Charlemagne was so impressed with the calming effect that the herb lemon balm had on his subjects that he ordered it planted at all the monasteries and medicinal gardens throughout his vast kingdom.

He helped make lemon balm available to the masses—and hundreds of years later, we know that lemon balm can be a powerful natural remedy for helping you get to sleep (and stay asleep).

Lemon balm is great for calming away stress, and in one double-blind, placebo-controlled study, people who took 600 mg of lemon balm daily reported feeling significantly less anxiety.

And in another international study, lemon balm extract helped relieve anxiety and reduce the number of sleep disturbances among patients. In fact, a whopping 95 percent of people responded to the treatment!

Lemon balm is thought to work by increasing the concentration of GABA, a key neurotransmitter that helps to promote sleep.

You can buy lemon balm extract as a stand-alone supplement. But it's often combined with other sleep-promoting natural ingredients like melatonin and L-theanine.

One truly effective multi-ingredient product is *Nature's Sleep Solution*, which is sold by Gold Leaf Nutritionals (a supplement supplier affiliated with the Alliance for Advanced Health).

You can get Nature's Sleep Solution risk-free at **www.goldleafnutritionals.com**.

Weird Blanket Stops Tossing and Turning in ONE NIGHT

On those cold winter nights, there's nothing better than snuggling under your favorite heavy blanket.

But if you find yourself restless and agitated at night—or are caring for someone who is—we're about to change what you consider "heavy."

Because there's a special type of heavy blanket—first popularized in nursing homes—that's been proven to calm night-time agitation fast.

It often works the very first night.

It's called a "weighted blanket," and it can weigh as much as 20 pounds. Weighted blankets typically use plastic or tiny glass pellets that are sewn into compartments.

These compartments ensure that the weight is consistent throughout the blanket.

Weighted blankets can provide relief from a variety of debilitating disorders (we will get deeper into these in just a bit) without the use of prescription drugs.

These special blankets seem to tap into something humans have used to induce calm since the start of our existence—being held.

Studies indicate that stimulating certain pressure points on the body can release serotonin, the chemical that helps regulate brain functions like mood and sleep. This is why the feeling of being held is so important.

Native Americans famously transferred this idea into a practice called swaddling. Many hospitals, birthing centers and parents continue the practice today.

Research has found that weighted blankets may have health benefits for older folks as well.

A study found that using a weighted blanket reduced the anxiety levels in 63 percent of the participants. This claim has been since supported by other papers.

Another study with participants who suffered from stress, pain and sleep issues showed that that when the subjects slept with weighted blankets, they experienced a reduction in cortisol. Reducing cortisol, which is the main stress hormone, can lead to better overall sleep quality.

In addition, weighted blankets have benefited folks with a variety of anxiety disorders, aggression, obsessive-compulsive disorder, ADHD and post-traumatic stress disorder with zero risk.

This means, this simple blanket could be a better solution than mind-numbing psychotropic pharmaceuticals for many folks.

A good rule of thumb when selecting the appropriate weight is 10 percent of one's body weight plus 1 pound.

Sensory Goods is a reliable manufacturer of weighted blankets. You can check them out at **www.sensorygoods.com**.

Japanese Farmer's Secret Makes Nighttime Anxiety Disappear

It's a sleep problem faced by millions of Americans today.

You know it's time to sleep—but your mind is racing with all the stresses and thoughts of the day, like a record player that keeps repeating.

If you have trouble calming down at night…if you have ever wished you could just turn off those anxious thoughts… the herbal remedy L-theanine is the answer you've been searching for.

And the story behind it is nothing short of a miracle.

You see, we all know how important tea is to Japanese culture. But did you know that 300 years ago, only the wealthiest Japanese nobility could afford it?

And that's when a simple Japanese farmer named Soen Nagatani changed his country…and rescued *you* from a lifetime of sleepless nights…*forever*.

He spent 15 years working day and night to develop a new type of tea that could be enjoyed by everyone. Japan even built a statue of him!

But when people started drinking his new "sencha" tea,

they noticed something amazing!

It was as if all their cares, stresses, and anxieties…like the ones that keep you up night after night…*just melted away.* Sounds good, right?

We know now that it's because of the miraculous, natural compound in the tea called L-theanine.

You see, L-theanine works to increase your brain's natural supply of GABA. That's a key neurotransmitter that actually calms the over-excited, stressed-out neurons in your brain.

It's the kind of calming action you can't…and *won't*…fall asleep without.

In fact, in an amazing study out of Australia, L-theanine was more effective at reducing stress and anxiety than the prescription drug Xanax—but without the risk of addiction or other terrible side effects.

In another study out of Japan, adults who took 200 mg of L-theanine reported sleeping better and feeling less exhausted the next day.

Imagine what it would be like for you to finally get the quality sleep you deserve—and to have the energy to tackle whatever each day throws at you.

With all the solid research behind L-theanine, it's practically a crime that mainstream doctors don't recommend it more for patients. Instead, they'll prescribe you heavy-duty "knockout" drugs that can leave you feeling like you have a hangover the whole next day.

But the good news is that you can get your hands on L-theanine easily enough. Piping Rock Health Products sells a 200 mg product (the same dose used in the Japanese study) for less than $10.

You can buy it at **www.pipingrock.com.**

5-Minute Bed Hacks Help You Sleep Longer and Better

When it comes to getting a good night's sleep, having the right bed is the first step.

We've all had the miserable experience of trying to sleep on a hotel bed—or a mattress at a friend's house—that didn't give us the rest and support we needed.

But believe it or not, there are some simple hacks you can make in your own bedroom. And they can go a long way toward giving you a better and deeper rest each and every night.

Hack #1: Raise your bed ends

Stack up a pile of pillows at the head of your bed, sloping them backwards, to support your back, neck and head in a raised position as you sleep.

This posture will aid digestion, making you feel more comfortable, and lift body weight off your heart and lungs, freeing up your breathing and circulation. With all these physical improvements, you'll find it much easier to relax.

Hack #2: Improve your mattress—without buying a new one

When it comes to picking a mattress, the Goldilocks Principle definitely applies—you're looking for firmness that's just right. A firm mattress will support your back, preventing muscle ache and joint pain.

But you want to avoid a mattress that's so hard that it's creating pressure points that will wake you up throughout the night. Before you donate that old mattress to Goodwill, there are some easy improvements you can make that may save you a bundle.

If you need to improve the firmness of your mattress, slide boards underneath it for support. If your mattress is too hard, try adding a duvet before buying a new one.

Hack #3: Position your bed for convenience

Where is your bed situated? If you're getting up every night to reach your lamp, water or other items, reposition your furniture so you can reach everything from your bed and avoid waking yourself up too much.

Check other logistics, too. Perhaps your bed is too far from the window, preventing the refreshing air from reaching you; or too near, causing a drafty feeling. Bright beams may also be keeping you awake. Cover up any distracting light sources, such as interior and exterior windows and monitor lights.

If your bed is in the middle of the room, how about pushing it into a corner for a cosier, more secure feel? A sense of security is another key sleep-inducer.

Hack #4: Try scented fabrics

Fresh, fragrant sheets can do wonders for inducing sleep. Next time you're shopping for washing detergent or conditioner, choose a scent that will calm and soothe you. In the coming pages, we'll also show you some effective aromatherapy tricks that can help you fall asleep.

Use Red Light and Pink Noise to Soothe Your Body to Sleep

There's one simple question that can make all the difference in determining whether you're getting all the sleep you need each and every night.

Is your bedroom just for sleep—or have you turned it into a den, with the latest flat-screen TV and other high-tech gadgets?

It's been proven that the light emitted by TVs, laptops and smart phones can interfere with your body's melatonin levels, fooling your brain into thinking it's the height of daytime rather than time for rest and sleep.

This is where the remarkable "red light trick" comes into play. You see, the light from electronic devices is so disruptive to sleep because it's strongly toward the blue end of the spectrum, much like the light from the sun.

So it's worth taking the opposite approach if you want to sleep. Fill your room with red light to mimic the natural composition of moonlight and give your body a strong hint that it's time for sleep.

Luckily, for this to be effective, you don't need a bright red neon sign in your room; an infrared lamp such as those found in the rodents section of a pet store will be fine, and will provide the right low-level red light ambiance to help you fall asleep.

The second trick relies on an incredibly effective sound called "pink noise." You may have heard of pink noise—it's a softer, slightly deeper version of the white noise produced by an old-fashioned detuned TV.

You've also probably seen white noise machines on the market.

Studies have found that when sleepers were exposed to pink noise, not only did they report a more restful sleep, but their brain activity was significantly decreased (which is critical for sleep).

A good source of pink noise is a simple electric fan, although there are also apps available for tablets and smartphones which produce a variety of pink noise effects, from breaking ocean waves to lulling raindrop sounds (just search for "pink noise" on your phone's app store). Just make sure your phone is facedown so you don't get any of its disruptive light.

Some lucky people can fall asleep almost at will. But if you're one of the many who find it more of a struggle, these two simple tips of red light and pink noise can make a real difference.

The Underground Secret to Perfect Sleep is Hiding in Your *Nose*!

When it comes to getting perfect sleep, scent is probably one of the last senses we think about.

We focus on sound, like disruptive noises...or even the touch and texture of our sheets and pillows.

But when it comes to catching some great Zs night after night, the answer may all come back to your nose.

Aromatherapy, the use of scents to promote better health, has been used successfully by traditional healers for thousands of years. It's natural, non-addictive (let's see those pricey sleep drugs make that claim) and doesn't come with side effects.

Better still, there are lots of different ways to use the therapy.

You can take a bath with a lavender-infused bath soak, try a scented pillow spray, or put an oil diffuser beside your bed.

So which essential oils should you use to improve your sleep?

Lavender is one of the most commonly used aromatherapy sleep aids as its scent is particularly pleasant, and it has been linked to relaxation and better sleep throughout the ages.

More recently, it has been shown to improve sleep and reduce anxiety in hospital patients and people with insomnia, so it is a good place to start if you're interested in herbal remedies.

Chamomile is another popular choice, particularly the sedative Roman chamomile essential oil.

Valerian, ylang ylang, cedarwood, and rose are all associated with enhanced relaxation and better sleep too and can be used in many soothing combinations.

Even sweet marjoram has been used as a sleep aid although some people find the scent objectionable.

Whatever your preference, there is an essential oil that can help. A reputable supplier of essential oils can be found at **www.aromatics.com**.

Is Your Brain's "Sleep Clock" Broken? Here's How to Fix It

If you've been struggling with sleep problems for years…and have been desperately searching for help…you probably know all about your Circadian Rhythm.

It's like your internal clock that tells your brain when it's time to sleep…and when it's time to wake up.

Well, you know what happens when the batteries die in one of your clocks at home, right? The clock says it's 3 in the afternoon when it's really 11 at night.

And, believe it or not, the *exact same thing* happens with your body's internal clock.

Your Circadian Rhythm…this powerful internal clock… depends on a constant supply of the natural hormone melatonin to work right. It's like a battery.

And that's a big problem, because the older we get, the less melatonin our bodies naturally produce.

Without enough melatonin, your brain actually can't tell the difference between day and night…and that's how you end up wide awake at 2 a.m.

The good news is that when you replenish your natural

supply of melatonin, your body's internal clock will spring back to life…and start working right…just like when you put new batteries into the clock at home.

One incredible study of more than 300 people who were aged 55 and older found that people who took melatonin fell asleep faster, slept better, and woke feeling more refreshed in the morning.

That just makes sense, right? With melatonin, you're finally giving your body the natural sleep support it's been *crying out for!*

And here's the best part—in another study published in the most prestigious sleep journal in the world, people who took melatonin got ***40 extra minutes of deep sleep every single night.***

Believe it or not, these were folks on heavy-duty high blood pressure drugs, which can make it nearly impossible to sleep. And the melatonin *still* worked!

So just imagine what 40 extra minutes of deep, peaceful sleep every night could mean for your energy levels…your concentration and focus…and even your health!

It's easy to start putting melatonin, this natural sleep hormone, to work for you. You can pick it up in capsule, liquid, or even lozenge form from NOW Foods at **www.nowfoods. com**.

CHAPTER 3:

THE DRUG-FREE SECRETS TO MAKING YOUR HEART (and Arteries) FEEL 10 YEARS YOUNGER

Dissolve Blood Clots (and Improve Your Heart) With This "Stink Custard"

Dealing with blood clots can feel a little like living on borrowed time. You know that just one bad clot can trigger a serious heart attack or stroke—or even cost you your life.

So how does the mainstream deal with the problem? They put you on prescription drugs that can be just as frightening.

In fact, one of the most prescribed meds, warfarin, can even trigger uncontrollable bleeding that can turn deadly in a hurry.

But what if you could actually dissolve clots—and give your heart health a serious boost—*without touching prescription meds?*

Imagine how good you'd feel knowing you were taking care of a serious problem without putting your health…or even your life…in jeopardy.

This isn't science fiction or some promising development that's still years away. The truth is…

The Japanese discovered the natural secret to beating clots CENTURIES ago!

It's called nattokinase, and it's derived from a fermented soybean food called natto that the Japanese have been eating since the Middle Ages. Some people aren't fans of natto's taste or smell, and it's even been called "stink custard" (but you don't have to eat it…more on that in a moment).

Science has shown that nattokinase is a clot-busting break-through…one that many patients like you are never told about.

In one study out of Japan, researchers found that once patients ate natto, the time it took for clots to dissolve was cut in HALF!

And in another study, 12 men were given either a dose of nattokinase or a placebo. Then their blood was drawn at 2, 4, 6, and 8 hours.

Just ONE DOSE of nattokinase was enough to reduce several of the blood markers for clots, including Factor VIII, a major blood-clotting protein.

Nattokinase may even stop deadly strokes!

Scientists in Japan even decided to see if nattokinase could help stop one of the deadliest clots around—and the results were jaw-dropping.

In an animal studies, researchers created carotid artery clots. Carotid arteries actually supply blood to our brains—and carotid artery disease is actually responsible for about half of all strokes every year.

But nattokinase was able to restore 62 percent of normal blood flow—which can mean the difference between life and death.

The clot-busting powers of nattokinase are literally saving and changing lives. Just look at the story of Mike, a 58-year-old man.

Mike had a bad clot in his retina, which was causing fluid buildup and bleeding. In fact…

He was slowly going *blind*…until he started taking nattokinase.

After just 20 days on nattokinase, Mike's vision had returned. And within two months, his clot had **completely dissolved**!

If all nattokinase could do was dissolve clots, it would still be one of the most powerful natural treatments around. But nattokinase also could hold the secret to naturally lowering your blood pressure, too!

In one study, patients with high blood pressure took 30 g. of natto extract a day. And they…

Lowered their blood pressure nearly 11 percent— in JUST 4 DAYS!

Just picture being able to control your blood pressure without having to resort to all those risky drugs. Some of those meds, like ACE inhibitors, have been linked to fatigue, dizziness, headaches, and even a swelling of your throat that can turn deadly.

And that's just the short list!

In fact, in one case study, published in the *Annals of Pharmacotherapy*, a 66-year-old man on ACE inhibitors died from severe throat swelling after taking the drugs. His doctors tried everything they could to save his life—but the problem was so severe that even epinephrine, antihistamines, and corticosteroids wouldn't work.

It's amazing that with all the risks that come with prescription drugs, more patients aren't offered safe, natural treatments like nattokinase. But blood pressure meds and anticoagulants are big business for Big Pharma—and they'll do everything they can to keep these safer remedies in the shadows.

But you shouldn't have to wait for mainstream medicine to

see the light. You can start putting nattokinase to work for you today.

The best way to get nattokinase is in supplement form. You can buy Doctor's Best Nattokinase at **www.iherb.com**.

But a word of caution—don't take nattokinase if you're already on blood thinners, as it can intensify the blood-thinning effect of the drugs.

The Jesuit Priest's Secret to Perfect Circulation

Do your hands and feet always seem to be cold? Even when the thermostat is turned way up?

Or do they ever get a "pins and needles" tingling sensation that doesn't seem to go away, no matter what you try?

These can both be symptoms of poor circulation. And it's more than just a nuisance—it can actually be an indicator of a more serious heart issue, and over time it can lead to permanent nerve and tissue damage.

Luckily, there's now an easy way to improve your circulation in as little as *30 minutes flat*.

And we may have a 17th century Jesuit priest to thank for it.

This miracle circulation booster is the lychee, a type of berry that grows in certain regions of China.

The Jesuit missionary Michael Boym was so intrigued by lychees—which are considered a symbol of romance and love in China—that he brought them back to Europe with him in 1656.

And once scientists started digging into the health benefits of lychees, they ended up falling in love, too.

It turns out the nutrients in lychees make them a heart-health superfood. They're low in sodium and high in fatty acids, which are great for your heart.

Plus, they're loaded with antioxidants that help them prevent oxidative damage to your heart, arteries, and just about everywhere else in your body.

But it's lychees' ability to improve poor circulation that's really turning heads in the alternative health community.

In a small study out of Japan, researchers tested a lychee extract on men and women with poor circulation to their extremities. Then they used a type of heat sensor to measure blood flow to the neck, shoulders and palms.

And what they discovered was *amazing*! The lychee extract started improving circulation in just 30 minutes!

In fact the best results were in the patients' hands, which are often a major circulation trouble spot.

Better circulation in 30 minutes—all thanks to a delicious fruit that people have been enjoying for ages.

And in another study on athletes, researchers found that lychee extract significantly reduced inflammation, which can be a major risk factor for heart disease.

But, believe it or not, that's not all lychees can do. They're also a rich source of natural phenols, which are chemicals that can inhibit some enzymes that promote cancer.

Lychees are a bit of an exotic fruit, so getting your hands on them can be tough (although more natural foods stores are carrying them).

The good news is that you can pick up Genceutic Naturals Lychee Superfruit supplements (500 mg.) at **www.vitadigest. com**.

Told Your Congestive Heart Failure Was Irreversible? Try This!

If you or someone you love suffers from congestive heart failure (CHF), it can feel like the bad news never stops coming.

You've probably had doctors tell you that the condition only gets worse...that it's incurable...and that it's probably going to shorten your life.

And there's a good chance you're being loaded up with diuretic drugs that can leave you dizzy, constantly cramping, and running to the bathroom non-stop.

CHF is a condition where your heart gets weaker and weaker, to the point where it can no longer pump blood effectively. You end up with shortness of breath, fatigue, and even major fluid buildup in your limbs.

And it's true that if you don't treat CHF effectively, it can cause lots of suffering and shave years off your life. But the good news is that there are natural supplements that can help alleviate even the most serious CHF symptoms.

And these natural remedies may hold the key to getting your CHF under control and improving your quality of life.

CHF Remedy #1: CoQ10

One of the most powerful nutritional supplements recommended for people experiencing heart failure is CoQ10 (we'll be talking more about CoQ10 later in this chapter). This substance is found in all our body cells and is a major energy source—but as we age, the amount of CoQ10 that our bodies produce decreases drastically.

Several studies have shown that CoQ10 increases the ejection fraction in heart failure patients. This is a measure of the amount of blood the heart can force out with each contraction.

Patients with congestive heart failure may benefit by taking 100 to 300 mg of CoQ10 each day, depending on the severity of the condition. CoQ10 is fat soluble, so it should be taken with meals.

You can buy Doctor's Best High-Absorption CoQ10 in 100 mg. capsules at **www.vitacost.com**.

CHF Remedy #2: Taurine

Taurine is an amino acid that can help the heart beat more forcefully. Supplemental taurine can help reduce the buildup of fluids in the body, thus lessening the workload of your weakened heart. A dose of two to six grams a day may be beneficial for CHF patients.

You can pick up taurine supplements affordably at **www.pureformulas.com.**

CHF Remedy #3: L-carnitine

L-carnitine can be helpful for people experiencing heart failure because it helps the cells in the body create more energy. It does this by transporting fatty acids inside the cell where they can be metabolized to produce energy.

Since the heart requires a lot of energy in order to function, one to three grams a day can help to make the heart stronger.

You can also pick up L-carnitine supplements at **www.pureformulas.com.**

CHF Remedy #4: Vitamin B1

In some patients, heart failure is related to a deficiency of vitamin B1, or thiamine. This deficiency is especially common in people who are alcoholics.

A daily supplement of 50 mg. of thiamine should be taken as part of a balanced vitamin B complex. You can pick up a B complex easily enough at most supermarkets or pharmacies.

Weird Potato Sinks High Blood Pressure Like a Stone

If you're on a restrictive diet, you've probably been told for years to avoid starchy foods.

And there's a good chance that potatoes are pretty high on your doctor's "naughty list."

But if you have high blood pressure, that advice could be wrecking your health.

Because research has now proven that these forbidden "potatoes" may hold the key to dropping your blood pressure and giving your heart health a major boost.

But there's one major catch—you have to eat the right potatoes.

A study published in the *Journal of Agricultural and Food Chemistry* found that eating purple majesty potatoes can lower high blood pressure without causing weight gain.

Now if you haven't had purple majesty potatoes before, you're not alone. They're kind of the weird ugly duckling of the potato family—they have dark purple skin and bright purple flesh.

They were first cultivated in Colorado as part of a push to

develop potatoes with more antioxidants and nutrients.

And now we're learning that the purple majesty potato may be the next great heart superfood.

For the study, 18 people ate six to eight small potatoes, including the skins, twice each day for one month.

While that may sound like a lot of potatoes, they were only about the size of golf balls.

And the potatoes weren't just delicious—they started dropping patients' blood pressure, too.

Study participants experienced an average reduction in diastolic blood pressure of 4.3 percent and in systolic pressure by 3.5 percent.

While that may not seem like much, keep in mind that blood pressure reductions (even on medications) don't tend to be dramatic. And these reductions may be enough to drop high-normal blood pressure into the normal range.

Better still? Although eating potatoes is often said to cause weight gain, none of the 18 study participants—all of whom were overweight—gained weight during the research.

The study's lead researcher, Joe Vinson of the University of Scranton in Pennsylvania, used purple majesty potatoes because the purple pigment is particularly high in healthy phytochemicals that have been shown to help fight lots of different diseases.

Its phytochemical content is actually similar to broccoli and spinach, which are already considered nutrient-rich superfoods.

Purple majesty potatoes are starting to become available in more grocery stores, particularly those that carry more unusual items. You also may be able to find them at farmers' markets.

The cooking method is important, because the high cooking temperatures involved with deep frying seem to destroy most of the beneficial nutrients in all kinds of potatoes.

If you have trouble finding purple majesty potatoes locally, you can actually grow your own. You can buy tubers for growing at **www.burpee.com**.

Slash Your Heart Risk By Eating MORE Fried Foods?!?

Let's face it—there's nothing better than biting into a fried chicken drumstick or a piping-hot onion ring.

But if you're like most folks, it's probably been a while since you had the sensation of grease dripping down your chin.

There always seems to be a spouse, child, or doctor waiting in the wings to warn you about the dangers of fried foods.

But what if everything...and we mean EVERYTHING... we've been told about fried foods is wrong?

A recent study reveals that our trusty frying pan may not be nearly as dangerous as we thought.

And enjoying fried foods the *right way* may be the key to keeping your heart in tip-top shape.

Research from the University of Edinburgh shows that the problem with fried foods isn't the grease at all—unless it's too hot.

It turns out that cooking foods at temperatures higher than 300 degrees F (150 C) changes their chemical structures.

That can lead to the formation of toxins called neoformed contaminants (NFCs).

This can get a little complicated, but here's what you need to know. NFCs include trans fat, which are notorious heart-wreckers (think nasty stuff in margarine), and glycogen end products that increase your risk for heart disease.

Foods fried at high temperatures are particularly dangerous because the oils rapidly break down and form trans fats.

Plus, the danger increases when cooking oils are reused (like at your favorite fast-food dive). Each use ups the amount of trans fats and your risk of heart troubles.

That's the bad news. The good news is that frying foods at lower temperatures may not be unhealthy at all...it can even be good for you.

To prove this, an international team of researchers scoured past studies that focused on how NFCs affected the heart health of both humans and animals.

Then they looked at heart disease rates in certain countries around the world.

People from South Asian countries like India, Bangladesh, Pakistan, and Sri Lanka, where foods are deep-fried at high temperatures, were FOUR TIMES as likely to suffer from heart disease.

But nearby China had the lowest risk of heart disease. The researchers think this is due to Chinese meals having more foods that are lightly fried at lower temperatures.

And, of course, we know that frying foods can actually be GOOD for your heart. That's because some cooking oils like olive oil and coconut oil come with plenty of heart-friendly benefits.

A good rule of thumb is to make sure the fried food you eat comes from your own kitchen, and not some burger joint or greasy spoon diner. This is the only way to be sure the cooking oils aren't being used repeatedly.

Second, never fry your foods at temperatures higher than 300 degrees F. And while that sounds low, it works just fine for delicious fried chicken.

Could ONE Supplement Keep You from *Ever* Having a Heart Attack Again?!?

If you've ever suffered a heart attack, you probably made a promise to yourself a long time ago.

Never again.

No more rides in the back of an ambulance. No more being wheeled into an operating room while your life hangs in the balance.

But there's a good chance that your cardiologist has told you that once you've had a heart attack, you're at greater risk for another one.

The bad news is that he's right. The good news is that this doesn't have to be your fate at all.

Because scientists have discovered that one breakthrough supplement may prevent you from ever having another heart attack again. And getting your hands on it couldn't be easier (if you know where to look).

This miracle discovery is CoQ10, the powerful enzyme we talked about a bit earlier in this chapter. And if you've had a heart attack, it's time to incorporate CoQ10 into your supplement regimen—right away.

CoQ10 is a fuel used for energy by our bodies' cells—and your heart's cells are in desperate need of an energy boost after a heart attack.

In a study out of India, one group of patients was given CoQ10 after a heart attack, and the other group was given a placebo.

And after just 28 days, the results were miraculous.

The patients taking CoQ10 were nearly **two-thirds less likely** to suffer angina and poor function of their hearts' left ventricles.

And episodes of heart arrhythmias were cut by more than HALF!

Again, that's after just 28 days!

And here's the best part—the people taking CoQ10 were less than half as likely to suffer another heart attack or die during the study!

The researchers recommend that heart patients start taking CoQ10 within three days after a heart attack—but research has also shown it may help you recover better if you take it before heart surgery.

And the benefits of CoQ10 go way beyond preventing heart attacks. One study showed it can even protect your heart from damage from chemotherapy.

Plus, CoQ10 can lower blood pressure and may even help you better control your blood sugar.

You can buy Doctor's Best High-Absorption CoQ10 in 100 mg. capsules at **www.vitacost.com**.

World War II Discovery Prevents Heart Death (and the Government Was FORCED to Admit It)

If there's one thing the government hates, it's having to admit that alternative therapies…ones that don't involve prescription drugs or risky surgeries…work.

But Uncle Sam is eating a lot of crow these days.

Because the government's own research has now confirmed that a powerful therapy being used by countless alternative docs…one that was first discovered during World War II…can stop heart attacks and deaths.

But these same government scientists are now doing everything they can to keep this breakthrough treatment out of your hands.

It's called chelation, and it's the process of injecting you with compounds (known as chelating agents) that bind to and remove toxins (especially heavy metals) from your body.

And the story behind chelation is like something right out of a spy novel.

If you remember your history, you know that during World War I, both sides bombarded each other with chemical weapons. You've probably seen the pictures of soldiers in gas masks as ominous chemical clouds hung above their heads.

Well, the British were worried that the Germans were going to try the same thing during World War II. So they asked a team of Oxford scientists to develop a life-saving treatment that could pull toxins out of soldiers' bodies.

The scientists succeeded—and that's how chelation was born.

Fortunately, there didn't turn out to be much need for chelation during World War II. But it was put to use in the United States soon after.

In fact, this therapy was used to save the lives of U.S. sailors who had developed lead poisoning painting ships for the Navy.

Alternative doctors have now been using chelation for decades to help remove toxins that have been linked to everything from neurological conditions to diabetes to heart disease.

The treatment was getting such positive results that the federal government even kicked in some money to study it (or debunk it…more on that in a moment).

They launched a study called the Trial to Assess Chelation Therapy (TACT)—and it produced results that these government scientists were never expecting.

In fact, the government's own research *proved* that chelation may prevent you from having a heart attack or dying from heart disease.

The patients in the study who received chelation treatments were an impressive 12 percent less likely to suffer from what were considered serious, negative "endpoints," like a heart attack, stroke, hospitalization for angina, or death.

But here's the *really* good news.

The patients with diabetes were a whopping **34 percent less likely** to have a serious heart episode or death. And you know that heart disease is a major complication that often comes with diabetes.

One-third less heart risk, using a proven treatment that's been around for decades. You would have thought our government would have been recommending chelation to diabetics everywhere.

Well, not exactly.

In fact, the study's authors said the results were "unexpected" and called for additional research.

Unexpected?!? In other words, these government researchers practically *admitted* the goal of the study was for chelation to fail.

It's just more proof that our government will do anything it can to try to downplay the effectiveness of alternative treatments—even when our government's own research proves these treatments work.

The government and mainstream medicine may be under the spell of powerful drug companies and their lobbyists, but you don't need to be.

There are plenty of places you can get chelation. You'll sometimes see it called EDTA chelation, as ethylene diamine tetra-acetic acid is a very common chelating agent and the one that was used in the government research.

To find a doctor near you who offers chelation, use the physician finder on the American College for Advancement in Medicine website (**www.acam.org**). It's under the "Resources" tab.

Delicious Dinner BLASTS Clogged Arteries

If you have plaque building up in your arteries, you've probably been told it's a ticking time bomb.

And it's one that could have you on the fast track to a heart attack or stroke.

But before you let some surgeon fit you for a stent, there's something you'll want to try first.

Because researchers have found a dead-simple menu formula you can enjoy any day of the week.

It features three of the most delicious foods around—and it could hold the secret to keeping your arteries healthy and clear.

For this latest study, the researchers tested a combination of omega-3 fatty acids found in oily fish, flavonols found in cocoa powder and dark chocolate and phytosterols found in nuts in a laboratory model.

And that's when they made a groundbreaking discovery…

By combining their active ingredients, these foods seem to stop the natural processes that lead to atherosclerosis, or hardening of the arteries. And they may help keep your arteries free of dangerous plaque.

This means by simply eating a meal that contains fish, dark chocolate (that's real chocolate, not the supermarket candy aisle junk) and nuts can help to keep your heart healthy and arteries clear.

What an easy formula to remember: Fish + dark chocolate + nuts = a healthy heart.

So put this formula to work—make a salmon dish for dinner and follow it up with a handful of decadent dark chocolate-covered nuts.

If that doesn't do it for you, try some pistachio-crusted tuna for dinner and a flourless chocolate torte for dessert.

Or if you're not a fan of fish, you can always supplement your omega-3s with a high-quality fish oil and still have dark chocolate-covered nuts for dessert.

Bottom line, it doesn't matter how you get these delicious and nutritious foods into your diet, just be sure you're enjoying them together.

10 Foods That Stop Inflammation COLD

It's the latest buzzword in medicine today—inflammation.

And with good reason. Inflammation is your body's natural response when it comes across allergens or unhealthy toxins.

It causes the release of immune cells and other compounds that are meant to deal with the threat.

And while that may sound like a good thing, many of us are in a constant state of inflammation thanks to the unhealthy foods we eat or even the nasty chemicals throughout our homes.

And over time, inflammation can cause cell damage and trigger serious health conditions—including heart disease.

Fortunately, there are plenty of tasty foods you can eat that are proven to fight inflammation and even give your immune system a natural boost.

Here are the top 10 foods to eat that can help keep inflammation under control:

Inflammation Fighter #1: Oily fish

Oily fish, such as salmon, mackerel, tuna and sardines are high in omega-3 fatty acids. A study conducted by the University of Hawaii found that men who ate baked or boiled fish several times a week reduced their risk of heart disease by up to 23 percent compared to those who didn't eat fish.

Inflammation Fighter #2: Dark leafy greens

Adding dark, leafy green vegetables into your regular diet can help protect the body from pro-inflammatory molecules known as cytokines. Spinach, broccoli, kale, and collard greens are also packed full of vitamins and minerals that contain antioxidant properties, which help to protect your body against free radicals and repair the damage caused by inflammation.

Inflammation Fighter #3: Nuts

Almonds and walnuts are excellent anti-inflammatory foods. Almonds are rich in calcium and vitamin E, while walnuts contain omega-3 fatty acids and more than 10 different antioxidant phytonutrients and polyphenols that play a positive role in reducing inflammation. All nuts are rich in antioxidants, so snack on a handful of nuts when you're feeling hungry.

Inflammation Fighter #4: Berries

Blue and red berries are packed full of antioxidants that help to reduce one of the body's inflammation markers known as TNF-alpha. Blueberries, raspberries, blackberries, and strawberries contain anthocyanins that have an anti-inflammatory effect.

Inflammation Fighter #5: Soy

Beans contain anti-inflammatory compounds called phytonutrients, but soy also has the ability to help reduce the body's inflammation marker C-reactive protein, which is linked to coronary artery disease. Aim to add more tofu and edamame beans into your diet.

Inflammation Fighter #6: Your kitchen spice rack

Even small amounts of herbs and spices can pack a powerful anti-inflammatory punch. Turmeric has strong anti-inflammatory, antioxidant, antiviral and antifungal properties. Basil and oregano are rich in antioxidant phytonutrients.

Rosemary, thyme, cinnamon and cloves also contain potent anti-inflammatory properties. Think about adding more healthy herbs and spices to add a health-kick to your meals.

Inflammation Fighter #7: Mushrooms

Regular white button mushrooms are rich in vitamin D, which helps to boost bone strength and reduces the risk of cancer. Mushrooms also contain polysaccharides, phenolic compounds, and lectins that help to suppress production of pro-inflammatory molecules.

Research conducted at Arizona State showed that button mushrooms were more effective for helping to suppress levels of inflammation, as compared to their more exotic cousins, like shitake, oyster, enoki, or crimini mushrooms.

Inflammation Fighter #8: Green tea

Green tea has powerful anti-inflammatory properties due to the antioxidant flavinoids it possesses. Researchers have found that green tea can reduce the severity of arthritis by helping to block the production of pro-inflammatory molecules that cause joint damage.

Studies also indicate that green tea can play a role in reducing inflammation associated with liver disease, inflammatory bowel disease (IBD), and some types of cancer.

Inflammation Fighter #9: Garlic and onions

Some of the most pungent vegetables are known for their immune-boosting properties. Studies have shown that compounds in garlic can block the pathways that lead to inflammation in a similar way to NSAID pain medications like ibuprofen. Onions contain similar compounds to garlic, along with the anti-inflammatory phytonutrients quercetin and allicin.

Inflammation Fighter #10: Beetroot

Bright red beets have powerful antioxidant properties that reduce inflammation, as well as protecting your body against cancer and heart disease. Beets are high in natural dietary fiber, and contain plenty of vitamin C. They're also rich in betalains that provide antioxidant and anti-inflammatory benefits.

CHAPTER 4:

PROTECT YOUR PROSTATE WITH THESE *AMAZING* NATURAL BREAKTHROUGHS

Pee Like a Teenager Again with This Incredible African Bark

If you're dealing with prostate problems, nighttime can be a little like dancing the Hokey Pokey.

You've constantly got one foot in the bathroom, and one foot out.

The urge to pee can come on suddenly, waking you up several times a night. But sometimes just getting your stream started or fully emptying your bladder can be a real challenge.

The good news is that there's a simple, natural remedy that can help tame even the trickiest prostate.

And it comes from an amazing tree that traditional African healers have been using for centuries.

Pygeum, a supplement derived from the bark of the African plum tree, has been wowing scientists around the world in study after study. And it may be the next big breakthrough treatment for benign prostatic hyperplasia (BPH).

You see, pygeum is loaded with phytosterols that can actually calm the runaway inflammation that can make your prostate swell up like a balloon.

In one study out of Europe, men who took 50 mg. of pygeum

for two months experienced an amazing 40 percent reduction in prostate symptoms.

And the good news didn't stop there.

These same men were getting up one-third fewer times at night to pee. How wonderful would that be to finally get the sleep you need without your prostate calling the shots?

Even better, a massive analysis of 18 studies found that pygeum can improve peak urine flow by 23 percent.

So no more drips and dribbles—you could end up peeing like a fire hose again.

Pygeum is backed by dozens of studies—so why aren't more men with enlarged prostates being given it?

Well, in some countries they are. In fact, it's the most common treatment for BPH in France, and is used widely in Italy.

But in the United States, the drug companies and most mainstream doctors are interested in pushing drugs like Proscar, which can cause dizziness and even kill your sex drive.

You can pick up pygeum pretty easily as a stand-alone supplement at **www.pipingrock.com**.

But you'll also see it included in supplement formulations with other prostate-friendly ingredients like saw palmetto or beta-sitosterol.

Just make sure you're getting enough. Much of the research on pygeum has focused on doses that were no less than 50–100mg.

Don't Let This Prostate "Gold Standard" Ruin Your Life

It shows up like clockwork in your mailbox every year or two—that postcard reminding you it's time for your prostate-specific antigen (PSA) test.

We've been told that the PSA is the "gold standard" for detecting prostate cancer early. We've even heard how it could save our lives.

But there's a whole lot more to the PSA story. And in many cases, skipping the PSA may save you a lifetime of pain and misery.

First, it's important to understand what the PSA is—and what it's not. The PSA is NOT a cancer test. It's a blood test designed to tell your doctor whether he should investigate further and maybe order a biopsy.

The problem is that the PSA test is wrong all the time. Simple things like BPH or an enlarged prostate can raise your PSA score. The next thing you know, you're getting a painful biopsy for nothing.

In fact, a study out of Canada found that as many as 20 percent of guys who basically "fail" their PSA test end up with a false-positive diagnosis. They don't have cancer at all—but they end up going through a lot of pain and anxiety before they find that out for sure.

And because the PSA test over-diagnoses cancer and is so unreliable, a lot of guys end up getting treatment they don't need.

Even when a PSA test eventually leads to a cancer diagnosis, lots of times it's a very slow-growing tumor that will never threaten your life. But mainstream doctors just can't help themselves—they'll zap it with radiation and try to cut it out.

The next thing you know, your sex life is ruined or you're wearing adult diapers.

"Some people believe men should be screened for cancer with the PSA test, but the evidence indicates otherwise," said Dr. Neil Bell, who works on a Canadian government task force.

Of course, there's big money in the PSA test, so most mainstream doctors want you tested early and often. In fact, the American Cancer Society wants some guys tested as early as 40.

But lots of scientists who look at the data will tell you that's nonsense. Even the American College of Physicians says lots of guys between the ages of 50-69 probably don't need the test, because the outcomes aren't any better for guys who get it.

Instead, they recommend discussing the PSA test's limitations with your doctor.

And as useless as the PSA test is, it's of even LESS value to men over 70, researchers say.

The Baseball Player's Secret to Beating Prostate Cancer

If baseball is America's pastime, then for a long time chewing tobacco was just about every baseball player's pastime.

It used to be that you couldn't watch a major league game without seeing just about every player with his lip packed full of the stuff.

That's died down a lot, and plenty of players moved to sunflower seeds instead. But now, more and more dugouts are featuring giant bags of pumpkin seeds, too.

And, believe it or not, lots of baseball players may have healthier prostates to show for it.

There's emerging science proving that pumpkin seeds may be the next big treatment for keeping prostate cancer and enlarged prostates in check.

Believe it or not, in the early 1900s pumpkin seeds were actually a pretty common treatment for enlarged prostate. Of course, that's before the drug companies became billion-dollar powerhouses and started taking over the medical industry.

Luckily, there have been scientists who haven't stopped investigating the wonders of pumpkin seeds.

In fact, a 2016 lab study out of Austria found that pumpkin seed extract can actually inhibit the growth of prostate cancer cells and cells from other types of cancer.

Another study on Korean men with BPH found that pumpkin seed extract significantly reduced prostate symptoms after only 3 months. The men were taking 320mg. a day.

Research out of Japan also found that pumpkin seed extract helped guys get up less at night to pee. And here was a real shocker—pumpkin seed extract has also been found to reduce episodes of incontinence in women.

So what's the secret here? Well, we know that pumpkin seeds are rich in zinc, which is important for prostate and bladder health.

But pumpkin seeds also have a good supply of antioxidants, which can be powerful weapons against inflammation and even cancer.

And the good news about pumpkin seeds doesn't end there. Research has shown they may be helpful for promoting healthy blood sugar and cholesterol levels.

So why didn't we include pumpkin seeds on our list of prostate superfoods? Well, there's a very good reason.

Your best bet, as far as pumpkin seeds are concerned, is to buy the extract as a supplement. You can get supplements in liquid or capsule form at the same (or greater) dosages that were used in studies, sometimes for less than $8 a month.

That makes pumpkin seed extract a smart option for guys with prostate issues. As you know, over-treating your prostate can be a mistake—but lots of men don't want to sit around and do nothing.

Taking a daily pumpkin seed extract supplement may be a happy middle ground.

This 2-second Prostate Cancer "Test" Won't Cost You a Dime

We've talked about how inaccurate the PSA test is for prostate cancer, and how it can lead to false-positives and the misery of over-treatment.

But, believe it or not, there may be a simple, do-it-yourself test that can tell you quickly if you're at risk for the most aggressive type of prostate cancer.

It only takes 2 seconds, and it's completely free.

Are you ready for it?

Stop reading this for a moment, and take a look down at your belly. Are you carrying around a bunch of excess belly fat? That proverbial spare tire?

Believe it or not, that bulging belly isn't just making your pants tight. It could be warning you of a possible cancer risk.

A study out of Oxford found that every extra four inches on your waist line increases your risk of the most dangerous and aggressive type of prostate cancer by 13 percent.

So if you should be a 32-inch waist, and you're a 36 instead, that's an extra 13 percent of risk. And if you're carrying around a 40-inch waist, that's an extra 26 percent risk.

Again, most prostate tumors are very slow-growing. What makes this study particularly noteworthy is that researchers focused on the aggressive forms of the disease.

So what does a beer belly have to do with cancer anyway? Well, we've known forever that there's a link between obesity and cancer.

And carrying around too much weight can promote inflammation and hormonal changes that are linked to cancer.

The good news is that big belly can give you an early warning that may help you stop cancer before it starts. Try switching to a protein-heavy diet that cuts out carbs, like the Paleo or so-called "caveman diet."

That also means no gut-busting processed foods.

Limiting your carbs is an easy way to shed some quick pounds. And it just may turn out that you're lowering your cancer risk in the process.

Underground Tips for MIND-BLOWING Sex After Prostate Surgery

We've talked a lot about ways to prevent prostate cancer… and how to deal with it after a diagnosis.

But maybe you aren't one of the lucky guys. There are countless men who have already had radical prostate cancer surgery.

And if you're one of them, you know it can absolutely destroy your sex life. It can affect everything from your ability to get an erection to whether or not you can have an orgasm.

The good news is that sex after prostate cancer surgery is not a lost cause. In the sex section of this book, you'll learn about some remarkably simple treatments for erectile dysfunction.

But here are 3 other things you can do, starting today, to make sex easier (or more pleasurable) after prostate cancer.

Tip #1: Get your testosterone levels checked

Low-T is a common problem after prostate surgery. And for years doctors were afraid to treat guys who had cancer with testosterone therapy. But more and more research is proving it's safe, and it's now become much easier to find doctors who will get you on a testosterone replacement plan.

Tip #2: Have your doc monitor your thyroid and prolactin

Low levels of thyroid hormone—or high levels of prolactin, which is made by your pituitary gland—can negatively affect your ability to reach orgasm.

But, for whatever reason, many doctors don't take a close enough look that these hormones. Normalizing your thyroid hormone and prolactin levels can go a long way to improving your sex life after a prostatectomy.

Tip #3: Try this under-the-tongue trick

Taking the hormone oxytocin under your tongue 5 to 10 minutes before sex can also help you reach an orgasm. This is the "love hormone" that kicks in during sexual arousal. It comes in sublingual form, and you can get a prescription from your doctor.

DO NOT confuse it with the painkiller OxyContin, which can be incredibly dangerous and addictive, and has been linked to numerous side effects.

You should also be careful to avoid drugs that can kill your sex drive like antidepressants. And remember that putting on weight can kill your sex drive and ability to perform as well.

Unfortunately, weight gain after prostate surgery is fairly common.

Poison Your Prostate?!? Skip This CRAZY Treatment

If you've been diagnosed with prostate cancer, you know the mainstream treatments range from bad to worse.

They've made billions offering guys bad choices like chemo and radiation, surgery that can ruin your sex life, or dreadful hormone therapies.

Now, believe it or not, they've upped the crazy...

They want to inject you with deadly bacteria that puts over 19,000 people in the hospital every year with uncontrollable fevers and diarrhea so dangerous it could even kill you.

This deadly bacterium is called salmonella, and it's the leading cause of foodborne illness.

For this study, a selected strain was injected into mice. To prevent the mice from falling ill, scientists altered the strain to be harmless.

Except it's not...unless you consider genetically modified organisms to be harmless.

And if the thought of being injected with genetically modified bacteria isn't terrifying enough...it turns out it doesn't even cure prostate cancer.

You see, the researchers chose salmonella because it's sneaky. Strains of these stealthy bacteria are able to penetrate through cell walls and then replicate inside of them. This means salmonella can infiltrate cells and then take them over.

This is great news if the bacteria can specifically target cancer cells.

And it seems in this study, the GMO bacteria were partially successful in doing that—the mice that were injected with the altered strain showed a 20 percent decrease in prostate tumor size.

However, the dangerous bacteria *didn't eliminate the tumor or stop the growth of cancer cells.*

This means you're taking a big risk for a small payoff.

Even though these bacteria are classified as "harmless," that doesn't mean there couldn't be complications. Bacteria often mutate. If this happens, they can be hard to kill and could even take over your healthy cells.

Plus, humans aren't mice.

In some cases, results from mouse studies can often translate to humans. But there's a big problem with this one…

The mice used for the experiment were also genetically modified.

So there's chance that much of this experiment's success hinged on finely tuned genetic factors. Genes this specific could make it difficult to replicate these results.

Lots of times, the best solution is to not rush into a treatment at all.

Studies have shown prostate cancer is often slow-growing and overtreated. That's why even some mainstream docs are starting to recommend "watchful waiting," which sounds like a more logical suggestion than injecting yourself with deadly bacteria.

7 Superfoods That CRUSH Prostate Problems

The best way to stop prostate problems is to never develop them in the first place.

That's just common sense, right?

But while we get lots of advice on how to eat to keep our hearts, brains, and waistlines healthy, nobody ever talks about how your diet can affect prostate health.

For sure there are foods to avoid, like sugars, carbs, and processed foods that can pack on the pounds and boost your prostate cancer risk.

But there are also foods that can keep your prostate healthy and functioning well. And loading up on these foods can help you avoid a lot of misery down the road.

Here are 7 foods that you can easily incorporate into your diet to improve your prostate health and lower your disease risk:

#1: Sesame seeds

Sesame seeds are rich in zinc, and zinc is essential to a healthy prostate. In fact, studies have found that men with BPH and prostate cancer are often low on zinc. That's one of the reasons you'll often see zinc in prostate supplements.

#2: Salmon

Salmon is rich in omega-3 fatty acids, which help control inflammation, like the kind that can affect your prostate. And don't forget that inflammation has repeatedly been linked to everything from heart disease to cancer.

#3: Berries (the darker, the better)

Berries like blueberries, blackberries, and raspberries are loaded with antioxidants. That's critical, because antioxidants help battle free radicals and the type of oxidative damage that can lead to cancer.

#4: Brazil nuts

Brazil nuts aren't just a tasty snack you can munch on while watching the football game. They also come with a healthy supply of the mineral selenium. And research has found that selenium may play a role in preventing prostate cancer. Like zinc, you'll often see selenium in prostate supplement formulations.

#5: Beans

Beans, like black beans, are loaded with fiber, which is essential for good prostate health. The nice thing about beans is that they're really easy to add to just about any meal, from salads to meat dishes.

#6: Bell peppers

We've talked a bit about the importance of antioxidants when it comes to prostate health. Bell peppers actually contain more vitamin C, a powerful antioxidant, than any other vegetable. You can incorporate bell peppers into meals or just cut some up for a snack.

#7: Tomatoes

Tomatoes are a great source of lycopene, which gives them their bright red color. And studies have shown that lycopene may be critical to lowering your prostate cancer risk. You'll also see lycopene as a fairly common ingredient in prostate supplements, and it's also sold as a stand-alone supplement.

Forgotten Egyptian Cure ERASES Prostate Problems

Jumpstart Your Sex Life and Slash Nightly Bathroom Visits 70%

Nothing destroys your quality of life faster than prostate problems.

You can't perform in bed like you used to.

You're running to the bathroom 6 or 7 times every night.

And how much time have you wasted standing in front of the toilet, hoping…praying…that something comes out?

If that sounds like you, you're not alone.

By the time you reach your 70s, there's a 90% chance you'll be suffering from benign prostatic hyperplasia, or **BPH**.

And mainstream medicine is full of drugs that are supposed to whip your swollen prostate back into shape…even though they can leave you dizzy, cause headaches, and wreck your sex drive.

Thanks for nothing, right?

But fixing your prostate doesn't have to be so complicated-—or dangerous.

There's a powerful natural prostate remedy that's been used since ancient Egyptian times. It's been PROVEN to deliver 70% relief for even the worst BPH symptoms.

Most American doctors don't know a thing about it…some would say this cure has even been "forgotten" to time.

But I'm going to show you how to get your hands on it…starting TODAY.

The Ancient CURE for BPH

If you have BPH, you probably have learned more about your prostate than you ever wanted to.

Your prostate is located just below your bladder and surrounds the urethra on all sides.

Normally, your prostate is quite small—about the size of a walnut. So when it becomes inflamed over time, it puts enormous pressure on your urethra and your bladder.

That can interfere with your sex life, and leave you feeling like you have to urinate all the time. Of course, getting any urine to actually come out is a whole other issue.

So what causes the problem?

As you age, your levels of a hormone called dihydrotestosterone (DHT) increase. DHT stimulates cell growth and causes prostate enlargement and BPH.

If you want to get your sex life back on track…end those midnight bathroom runs…and get your urine flow up to speed again, you need to shrink your prostate down to size.

And that's EXACTLY what **rye grass pollen** does.

Rye grass pollen is a remarkable substance that can be extracted from common rye grass.

Ancient Egyptians were reportedly using it all the way back in the 15th century B.C.—but it's practically been forgotten by modern medicine.

Rye grass pollen contains beta-sitosterols that attack BPH

and your prostate problems in at least three different ways:

#1: Rye grass pollen relaxes the muscles in your urethra, making it easier to pee.

#2: This powerful supplement boosts the tone of your bladder muscles, so you won't always feel like you have to urinate.

#3: Rye grass pollen slashes inflammation and swelling, and prevents the growth of prostate cells.

Plus, rye grass pollen has been found to contain at least 21 prostate-healthy amino acids, as well as enzymes, coenzymes, sterols, minerals, trace elements, and all known vitamins.

It doesn't just control BPH—it can REVERSE the condition completely.

In fact, **rye grass pollen has a stunning 70% success rate in relieving BPH**.

It's even run circles around some of the most popular prescription drugs on the market.

Rye Grass Pollen Can Save You From Drugs—And Surgery!

One landmark study looked at 60 men who had the worst BPH you could imagine.

Their urinary flow was so bad, they were being scheduled for surgery.

Of course, that's before they started taking two rye grass pollen capsules twice a day.

Researchers monitored key BPH symptoms, like having to pee urgently, dribbling, and having trouble urinating. And the results were AMAZING.

At the end of the six-month study, **the patients given rye grass pollen saw a nearly 70% improvement in their BPH symptoms,** compared to the men who got a placebo.

And that's not all.

Another placebo-controlled study compared rye grass pollen with the popular prostate drug Tadenan.

It turned out that 78 percent of patients saw greater improvement taking rye grass polen than they got with Tadenan.

Rye grass pollen ran circles around the best drugs Big Pharma had to offer.

Another study found that nearly 70% of men slashed their nighttime bathroom visits after taking rye grass pollen.

What would fewer trips to the toilet…and more sleep… mean for you?

So why haven't you heard of rye grass pollen—and why has your doctor never mentioned it to you?

The fact is, drug companies control medicine in America, and they have ZERO interest in promoting natural cures.

All while countries all over the world–from Western Europe to Japan, Korea, and South America—consider rye grass pollen a registered pharmaceutical product called Cernilton.

How to Get Your Hands on Rye Grass Pollen

If you or a loved one is suffering from BPH, look into adding rye grass pollen to your daily routine immediately.

The alternatives are truly shocking—from pricey meds riddled with risks to invasive surgeries!

You can buy Rye Grass supplements from reputable companies like Swanson Vitamins. Just follow the dosing instructions and you should notice a difference quickly.

Additionally, there are some other easy things you can do to prevent and control BPH:

- Urinate when you first get the urge.
- Go to the bathroom when you have the chance, even if you don't have an urge.
- Avoid alcohol and caffeine, especially after dinner.

- Spread out your fluid intake during the day.
- Avoid cold and sinus medications which can worsen symptoms.
- Exercise regularly.
- Reduce stress.

With the right routine, you'll have BPH under control in no time—without the crazy expenses, risky drugs, or surgery!

CHAPTER 5:

SEND ENERGY LEVELS *THROUGH THE ROOF* WITH THESE NATURAL TIPS

Mythical Indian Berry Gets Energy Levels *Soaring*

If you suffer from excessive fatigue, getting out of bed in the morning can be the hardest part of the day.

And you've probably tried just about everything to boost your energy levels, from going to bed earlier to guzzling cup after cup of coffee.

And if nothing has worked for you, it may be that you've never really gotten to the real root of your energy problems.

Your poorly functioning adrenal glands may be leaving you in constant exhaustion—and relief may be just a few short weeks away.

Your adrenal glands are located right above your kidneys, and they're responsible for regulating your body's stress response and energy levels.

But just like any other part of your body, your adrenals can get worn out. That's especially true if you're dealing with a lot of stress and are forcing your adrenals to work overtime.

Some of the most common symptoms of adrenal fatigue include:

• Constant exhaustion or lethargy

- Depression
- Anxiety
- Increased difficulty managing stress
- Brain fog
- Low blood sugar

Supporting your adrenals is essential to keeping you energetic and alert when you need to be. Fortunately, thanks to an ancient Indian remedy, there's an easy way to make sure your adrenals get the fuel they need.

It's called ashwagandha, and it's made from the Indian ginseng plant. And it's been used for centuries in traditional Ayurvedic medicine to treat issues like fatigue.

Ashwagandha is an adaptogen, which means it's designed to help your body manage its stress response and normalize its natural processes.

And ashwagandha's effects on energy levels are nothing short of miraculous. Studies out of Asia have found that ashwagandha is so powerful that it can even improve energy among patients who are undergoing chemotherapy.

And if you have ever seen how chemotherapy can wipe someone out, you know how impressive that is.

In another study, it even significantly improved energy and endurance among elite cyclists. These are people in fantastic shape and who have plenty of energy to burn...and they STILL benefited from ashwagandha.

Aside from supporting your adrenals, scientists believe ashwagandha also helps with the production of red blood cells and hemoglobin, which you need to deliver energy throughout your body.

Ashwagandha was a big secret to Western medicine for a long time...but, luckily, the word is starting to get out.

You can find ashwagandha just about any place that sells supplements. Typical recommended dosages are 1,000mg. a day and up.

BRI Nutrition makes a 1,000 mg. ashwagandha supplement that you can buy at **www.jet.com**.

The 7 Energy Busters Hiding in Your Medicine Cabinet

The numbers are mind-boggling—the average senior citizen in America is taking five or more different prescription drugs.

And if you want to know why so many seniors are feeling weaker or more exhausted than ever, prescription drug use is as good a reason as any.

Mainstream medicine hands out these drugs like candy, telling us they're going to make us feel better. But the fact is, chronic fatigue is a major side effect for many of the most popular medications on the market today.

Here are 7 drugs that may be leaving you tired all the time. If you're taking any of them, schedule an appointment with your doctor to talk about alternatives.

You'll also find alternatives to many of these medications throughout this book.

1. Blood pressure meds:

Just about every blood pressure drug makes this list, from ACE inhibitors like Prinivil and Zestril, to "water pill" diuretics.

2. Statins:

You might know these cholesterol-lowering drugs by brand names like Crestor, Lipitor, or Zocor.

3. Antibiotics:

Fatigue is a common side effect for many antibiotics, possibly because they destroy the healthy bacteria in your gut. Your gut flora play a critical role in maintaining energy levels.

4. Antidepressants:

Fatigue and lethargy are major problems with antidepressant drugs, especially selective serotonin re-uptake inhibitors (SSRIs) like Prozac and Paxil.

Some people claim to feel like "zombies" on the drugs. That's especially ironic, as fatigue is a major symptom of the depression that the drugs are supposed to treat.

5. Antihistamines:

No surprise here, right? Antihistamines like Benadryl have been knocking people out for decades.

6. Proton-pump inhibitors (PPIs):

This one may come as a bit of a surprise. But these stomach acid-blocking PPIs like Nexium, Prevacid, and Prilosec can actually cause a magnesium deficiency that can result in major fatigue.

7. Benzodiazepines:

"Benzos" like Klonopin, Valium and Xanax, are prescribed for anxiety, muscle spasms, and even sleep. But they depress your nervous system, which can leave you feeling exhausted.

For years medical groups have been recommending against prescribing benzos to seniors, as they've been linked to everything from falls to memory loss. But they're still pretty widely prescribed.

Is a Secret Thyroid Disorder Sapping Your Energy? Take This Quiz

You wake up in the morning and you feel like you didn't sleep at all. You're sluggish throughout the day and have trouble concentrating.

It's just part of getting older, right? Well, maybe not. You could be one of the countless Americans suffering from a thyroid disorder.

And the worst part is that mainstream medicine is notoriously terrible at diagnosing these problems, which leaves people like you feeling sapped and miserable.

Located between your collarbones, your thyroid is a butterfly-shaped organ that regulates various hormonal processes in your body. And when your thyroid health is out of whack, it can take an enormous toll on your energy.

So do you have an undiagnosed thyroid problem? This quiz is a good place to start to find out.

Question #1: Do you have problems with sleep & energy?

An underperforming thyroid doesn't produce enough hormones for the muscles and cells; as a result, they don't get the energy they need. Fatigue is a common symptom of an underactive thyroid (hypothyroidism).

If your thyroid is over-performing (hyperthyroidism), the excess hormones can cause anxiety and a quickened pulse, which make going to sleep much harder.

Question #2: Do you struggle with concentration and clarity?

An imbalance of thyroid hormones can affect your brain and all your mental functions. With hypothyroidism, you're not producing enough hormones and that can cause a lowered mood or even depression.

A malfunctioning thyroid also leads to less serotonin in the brain, and that reduces the amount of joy you might feel from day to day. On the other hand, an overactive thyroid can hamper your ability to concentrate by making so many hormones that your body enters a hyperactive state.

Question #3: Do you feel unusually hot or cold?

When you have hyperthyroidism and your thyroid is overactive, your energy-producing cells will work much harder. As a result, you may end up feeling hot or start sweating.

Hypothyroidism has the opposite effect. The lowered activity in your body leads to less energy production, and makes it harder to generate heat and resist the cold. The next thing you know, you're constantly reaching for an extra blanket or turning up the thermostat.

Question #4: Do you experience sudden pain or numbness?

Because thyroid issues can affect the brain, they can affect the nerves and spinal cord. A lack of thyroid hormones leads to the nerves getting damaged; in turn, they may send signals for sudden tingles, numbness, or even pain.

Feet, hands, and limbs are common targets, but various muscles could also experience that pain.

Question #5: Have you had any unexplained weight gain or loss?

Even if you're getting enough exercise and eating properly, a faulty thyroid can wreak havoc on your weight. An overactive thyroid leads to constant hunger, but you burn off the calories fast and can start shedding pounds.

With an underactive thyroid, you might not have much of an appetite, but it's harder to deal with the calories you take in. That can lead you to pack on extra weight, even if you're not eating that much.

So what can you do to keep your thyroid healthy—without turning to prescription drugs or other barbaric mainstream treatments? Just flip to the next section, and you'll learn all about three amazing foods that can keep your thyroid in perfect working order.

Eat These 3 Superfoods for a PERFECT Thyroid

The food choices we make play a huge role in determining how healthy our thyroids are—and whether we have the energy we need to tackle each and every day.

Unfortunately, we're surrounded by processed foods and fast-food, drive-through junk that can destroy perfectly healthy thyroids.

The good news is that if you add these three superfoods to your diet, you can nourish your wheezing thyroid back to health.

Superfood #1: Seaweed

Iodine is essential for a healthy thyroid. But that's a big problem, because only a small portion of the iodine in table salt is available to our cells. And with everyone telling us to cut back on salt, we're sitting ducks for an iodine deficiency and thyroid problems.

The iodine found in seaweed and wild-caught fish is the most nutritious and easily absorbed by the body, so invest in some wild-caught salmon if you can, or check out the grocery store for a seaweed fix. The most well-known seaweed is nori, but there are plenty of options, including kelp, dulse, hiziki, and wakame.

Superfood #2: Coconut oil

Saturated fat has been demonized by the mainstream for years, but with coconut oil we're learning just how important it is. The lauric acid found in coconut oil has a similar composition to breast milk, making it easier to digest.

Once the lauric acid is metabolized by the mitcochondria of your cells, it is converted into monolaurin, a powerful antibacterial and antiviral chemical that fights many of the contributors to low thyroid, including candida overgrowth and oxidative stress.

Holistic doctors usually recommend starting out with just a couple teaspoons of coconut oil a day, and then working up to 2 or 3 tablespoons.

Superfood #3: Eggs

The mainstream has been dead wrong about eggs for years. The fact is, they're a nutritional powerhouse that can boost thyroid function.

The thyroid relies on the mineral selenium to regulate the activity of its two main hormones, T4 and T3. Two eggs deliver 60 percent of your daily need for selenium.

Eggs also are an excellent source of iodine and are high in amino acids, both of which are essential to supporting your thyroid.

Feeding your thyroid can be absolutely delicious. Toasted, chopped dulse seaweed adds a crispy, almost bacon-like texture to salads (and we all love bacon), while wakame can add crunchiness to salads. Whip up scrambled eggs and sprinkle dulse flakes on them if you're still feeling seaweed-shy.

Coconut oil is incredibly versatile. Mix it with cocoa powder, peanut butter, stevia, and a spoonful of honey for an addictive and guilt-free treat. Blend it into your morning coffee or smoothies, use it in cooking, spread it on bread in place of butter, or (for the brave-hearted) eat it straight off the spoon.

5 Cheap, Natural Energy Boosters You Can Start Using *Today*

It happens to all of us. You're feeling drained and run-down and you start reaching for those unhealthy pick-me-ups like sugar-packed sweets or cans of soda.

But there are much easier and healthy ways to send your energy levels into the stratosphere—and lots of them may be sitting in your home right now.

Whether you're constantly battling fatigue, or just need a little pick-me-up, these five sources of natural energy are excellent everyday choices. And none of them have caffeine or additives.

Energy Booster #1: Ginseng

Ginseng has been a go-to in Chinese medicine for thousands of years. It's a powerful herb that is quickly and easily digested.

And the best part? Ginseng has become much more popular in recent years, and can often be found on grocery store shelves as an extract, powder, or tea, or in its whole root form.

Ginseng seems to work in part by dilating blood vessels and increasing oxygen flow to your brain. It can provide you with an instant energy burst, or you can consume it daily as part of your regular diet to contribute to a more balanced energy flow.

You can pick up ginseng supplements affordably at **www.luckyvitamin.com.**

Energy Booster #2: Water

Kind of boring, right? But hydration is a very overlooked piece of the energy puzzle.

Your body uses water to keep up proper physical functions, including waste removal, joint lubrication, and sodium transport. When you're not getting enough, you're going to feel sore and worn down.

Obviously, drinking water often throughout the day is the easiest solution, but delicious, water-saturated vegetables and fruits such as cucumbers, peppers, and melons can help out, too.

Energy Booster #3: Kiwi

These small, furry fruits are really underrated for their nutrition and energy boosting properties. A single kiwi typically contains double the potassium of a banana, twice as much vitamin C as an orange, and two to three grams of fiber, all of which are important energy-providing nutrients.

The natural (and healthy) sugar in the kiwi provides an instant increase in energy, and the fiber helps to keep you feeling full.

Energy Booster #4: Tyrosine

Tyrosine isn't exactly a household name, but when it comes to feeling refreshed and alert, this amino acid is worth its weight in gold.

It's quickly absorbed by the brain, meaning you will feel

its effects right after consuming it, and you can find it in high doses in quite a few delicious, versatile foods, such as salmon, cottage cheese, and eggs. You can also get it in supplements for about $10 a month at **www.luckyvitamin.com.**

Energy Booster #5: Oats

Regularly including oats in your diet is one of the cheapest, easiest, and best ways to fight off fatigue. The protein, magnesium, and B vitamins contained in oats are all great at boosting short-term energy levels, while their high fiber content helps your body use its food supply at a healthy rate, keeping your blood sugar levels balanced and your appetite satisfied.

LIVE LONG & STAY GORGEOUS WITH THESE ANTI-AGING SECRETS

Is This Russian "Spy Pill" the Secret to Limitless Aging?

Imagine workout out at the gym or going for a walk around your neighborhood, when you notice something amazing.

You're not tired...or sore. In fact, you have enough energy to push yourself harder and farther than you ever thought possible.

This isn't fantasy. For decades, the Soviet Union produced athletes who seemed to defy physical limits—against the best competition in the world.

They smashed world records. They hauled in more Olympic medals in the 1970s than any other country on Earth.

And now we know why. Because in a secret Siberian lab, Soviet scientists had done the impossible. They had discovered...

The natural secret to superhuman aging and performance!

It's all perfectly legal—and now you can get your hands on this amazing breakthrough to battle aging, pain, fatigue, and even cancer.

This remarkable discovery is called Rhodiola rosea, and it

may be the greatest medical advancement to ever emerge from the Soviet Union.

You see, behind the Iron Curtain, the top Soviet researchers weren't just developing secret submarines and nuclear weapons. They were trying to create a superhuman race of athletes, scientists, and leaders who could perform at the very highest levels on the world stage.

And Rhodiola rosea was their secret.

Rhodiola rosea is a beautiful yellow flower that grows in some of the most inhospitable regions of the planet, like Siberia and high altitudes in the Alps. It was used by nomadic Siberian tribes for ages to help deal with the stress of living in one of the harshest climates on Earth.

And when Soviet military scientists began experimenting with Rhodiola rosea in the 1970s, they discovered something amazing.

It turns out that Rhodiola rosea is an "adaptogen," which means that it naturally helps your body deal with physical and emotional stress. That means it can help you perform longer and better—mentally and physically—under even the toughest conditions.

Studies have found that it actually decreases your heart rate during strenuous exercise, so you can exercise at a high level with less exertion.

The Soviets secretly began supplying their athletes, cosmonauts, and even politicians with this incredible herbal breakthrough. They found that their Olympic biathletes could shoot targets without their arms shaking—even at the end of long, grueling races.

For decades Rhodiola rosea was kept a secret. But after the Cold War ended, a Soviet scientists defected to the United States with all the research and revealed...

One of the greatest natural anti-aging breakthroughs...ever

The science behind Rhodiola rosea is positively jaw-dropping.

One study out of Russia, published in 2004, found that Rhodiola rosea protected muscle tissue from damage during exercise and significantly lowered levels of C-reactive protein, a key marker of inflammation.

And preventing muscle damage and inflammation are absolutely critical, especially if you want to stay active as you get older.

And in another double-blind trial, patients who took 200 mg. of Rhodiola rosea were able to exercise longer and harder without becoming exhausted.

But, of course, that's not all Rhodiola rosea can do. It also may hold the secret to...

Banishing brain fog and keeping your brain razor-sharp... at ANY age!

In a study on middle-aged adults and seniors, all 120 patients who took Rhodiola rosea experienced significant increases in mental performance after just 12 weeks!

That's a 100 percent success rate!

And in an Ivy League study published in 2015, Rhodiola rosea performed nearly identically to Zoloft for treating major depression—but with far fewer side effects.

In fact, *a whopping 63 percent of the Zoloft patients ended up reporting side effects!* Talk about a risky drug!

If all Rhodiola rosea did was improve performance, soothe depression, and boost your brain, that would be plenty.

But now scientists are proving that...

Rhodiola rosea can *destroy* cancer cells, and maybe even keep you or someone you love alive.

In a lab study out of the University of California, Irvine, scientists exposed bladder cancer cell lines to a Rhodiola rosea extract.

And that's when something amazing happened—the cancer cells literally started self-destructing through a process called autophagy. Meanwhile, the healthy, non-cancerous cells were unharmed.

In another lab study out of Poland, leukemia cancer cells were exposed to a high concentration of Rhodiola rosea for 72 hours.

And virtually NONE of the cancer cells survived. That's right—*countless cancer cells killed in just three days.*

There's going to be plenty more research on Rhodiola rosea as a cancer-killer. But there's really no reason to wait—especially when we know all about all the other amazing anti-aging benefits this natural remedy provides.

And while Rhodiola rosea was once a major military secret, it's no longer hard to get your hands on it.

You can buy Swanson Health Products 400 mg. Rhodiola rosea extract at **www.swansonvitamins.com**. Expect to spend $10–$20 for a month's supply.

Got Wrinkles? ERASE Them for 32 Cents a Day!

They say you're only as old as you feel.

But come on—who wants to *look* a day older than they are?

Unfortunately, those creases, laugh lines, and crow's feet we develop over time can get pretty hard to hide.

If you're like a lot of people, you've tried just about every wrinkle cream on the market. And you've learned they work about as well as a screen door on a submarine.

But now scientists have discovered a supplement that can help erase wrinkles from the inside.

And you probably have enough change in your couch cushions to afford it.

Researchers conducted a small study where they asked women to take a daily methylsulfonylmethane (MSM) supplement for 16 weeks.

And that was all the time it took for these women to see a real, noticeable difference in their skin.

MSM actually improved the function of genes that are responsible for healthy skin—including the prevention of wrinkles.

But that's not all. The women who took MSM also saw noticeable improvement in crow's feet, skin firmness, tone and texture.

And MSM won't just help you look younger—there's a good chance you're going to end up feeling younger, too. That's because MSM is one of the most studied joint supplements around.

In fact, you'll often see MSM in supplement formulations alongside other joint-care powerhouses like glucosamine and chondroitin.

But what you'll really love about MSM is the price.

It's widely available, and you can often grab a month's supply for less than $10 at retailers like **www.puritan.com**.

That means you may be able to improve your skin—and your joint health—for around 32 cents a day.

And that's an investment in yourself that's well worth making.

Give Father Time a Run for His Money with This "Master" Antioxidant

Believe it or not, there's a war going on inside our bodies right now.

And our cells are the front lines.

That's because from the food we eat to the air we breathe, we're constantly bombarded by toxins that wreak havoc on our cells.

And over time, these toxins can age us prematurely and make us sitting ducks for some of the deadliest diseases around.

That's the bad news. The good news is that there's a simple, natural substance that holds the key to stopping this toxic buildup and helping us give Father Time a run for his money.

It's called glutathione, and it's so powerful that it's been known as the "master antioxidant."

Glutathione fights oxidative stress and can even help our cells ward off damage from the toxins we are in contact with daily.

Unfortunately, our glutathione levels can take a nosedive as we get older, and problems like stress and illness can make the problem worse.

Fortunately, you can help your body make the glutathione it needs—and use it more efficiently—with help from a supplement called N-acetyl-cysteine (NAC).

NAC has been used in emergency medicine for years to help patients rapidly detoxify their bodies, including patients suffering from certain drug overdoses. But researchers from Oregon State say it also may be useful for helping with daily detox, too.

That's because NAC is actually an important precursor to glutathione. That means it can jumpstart your body's natural production of this important antioxidant.

And that's big news, because low glutathione levels have been linked over the years to common diseases of aging, like heart disease, dementia, and even cancer.

In hospitals, NAC is often used intravenously. But you can also pick up NAC supplements from Biotics Research at **www.pureformulas.com** for around $30 a month.

That's an easy way to give your body a fighting chance against all those nasty, disease-causing toxins that can be hard to avoid.

90% of Women *Rave* About This Natural Hair-Loss Breakthrough

You've tried the wigs…and the hats…and the comb-overs… and even those "thickening" shampoos.

If you're a woman suffering from hair loss, odds are you've tried just about everything.

And you know that hair loss isn't just a physical problem that comes with age—there are plenty of emotional scars, too.

But now there's a natural cocktail that may help you win the battle against hair loss for good.

And you won't believe how well it works.

In a study published in 2015, women with thinning hair who took fish oil, blackcurrant seed oil, vitamin E, vitamin C, and lycopene every day for 6 months saw amazing results.

More than 60 percent experienced thicker hair, and 90 percent reported a decrease in hair loss.

What else on the market today is getting results like that?

Now, we've known for ages that some of these supplements like fish oil and vitamin E are essential for nourishing hair and keeping it healthy.

But researchers say this cocktail also goes to work on problems like inflammation, which can contribute to hair loss.

I know what you're thinking—that's an awful lot of supplements to take. But just consider how much time and money you've spent trying to cover up your hair-loss problem instead.

Here are the exact doses that were used in the research:

Fish oil: 460mg

Blackcurrant seed oil: 460mg

Vitamin E: 5mg

Vitamin C: 30mg

Lycopene: 1mg

You can pick up all these supplements at **www.puritan. com** or **www.luckyvitamin.com**.

Two quick things to remember—first, as with any supplement regimen, you want to make sure you give it enough time to work.

Second, if you haven't already, it's a smart idea to discuss any hair-loss issues with your doctor. You want to make sure there isn't a more serious issue, like an autoimmune reaction, occurring.

The 20-Minute Secret to Living to 100 (and You *Don't* Have to Diet)

These are supposed to be the best years of your life.

You know, time to kick back and enjoy yourself a little, right?

So why is everyone constantly giving you advice that makes you miserable?

They'll tell you that if you want to stay healthy and live longer, you need to give up all your favorite foods…go to bed early…or spend hours sweating away at the gym.

Adding years to your life shouldn't be that hard—and maybe it doesn't have to be.

Because researchers have discovered that the secret to living to 100 and beyond may be as simple as popping a vitamin or taking a 20-minute walk outside.

Scientists from the Buck Institute for Research on Aging have completed a jaw-dropping study on the life-extending powers of vitamin D, the "sunshine vitamin."

Worms that were given a daily supply of vitamin D actually lived a whopping 33 percent longer than their creepy-crawly pals who didn't get the vitamin.

Can you imagine what 33 percent more life could mean for people like you and me?

Now, I know what you're thinking—it's hard to get too worked up about a study on worms.

But, actually, worms are used all the time in both drug and supplement research. Because of their shorter life spans, we can learn how they react to things much more quickly.

And the idea that vitamin D can add candles to your birthday cake is just common sense. We've known for years that it can decrease your chances of Alzheimer's, diabetes, and even caner.

Our bodies can produce vitamin D naturally from the sun, so it's a good idea to spend at least 20 minutes a day outside with your head and arms exposed.

But if you live in a colder climate, it may be tough to get enough sunlight this time of year.

The good news is that you can pick up vitamin D supplements affordably at just about any supermarket or pharmacy.

Make Varicose Veins Disappear with This Old "Butcher's Remedy"

We all like to throw on our favorite pair of shorts in the nice weather, or strut around confidently in our swimsuits at the beach.

But if you have those unsightly blue varicose veins protruding all over your legs, you know how embarrassing they can be.

Varicose veins aren't just a nuisance—they can indicate a more serious issue where your veins aren't working like they should and blood is pooling (especially in your legs).

Of course, mainstream medicine is just waiting with expensive and uncomfortable surgery promising to zap those varicose veins away. Good luck getting your insurance to cover that!

Fortunately, there's a time-tested herbal remedy for varicose veins that most people have never heard about (the mainstream wants to sell you surgery, after all). And it could help make those blue spider webs disappear and improve your circulation.

It's called butcher's broom, and it's a spiny bush that grows all over the Mediterranean. And butchers once used its branches to help sweep the scraps off their floors.

But that's not all that butcher's broom is good for! It's been used in alternative medicine for ages to help treat everything from hemorrhoids to gallstones. And it may be the best weapon around for varicose veins.

That's because research has shown that butcher's broom can constrict your blood vessels, improve circulation, and work to prevent blood from pooling in your veins. It's been tested time and time again in around 30 clinical studies.

A study out of Germany found that butcher's broom worked wonders for improving vein function, when compared to a placebo—and without all the side effects that often come with prescription drugs.

Research has also shown butcher's broom can decrease that tell-tale swelling in your veins—one study out of Mexico found it significantly decreased swelling in the legs in just 12 weeks.

The typical recommended dosage of butcher's broom is at least 150 mg. a day. You'll often see it combined with other natural treatments for decreasing varicose veins and improving vein health, like horse chestnut.

You can find NOW Foods 200 mg. butcher's broom online at **www.pureformulas.com**.

Those Rough Fingernails Are a Canary in the Coal Mine! Here's How to Fix Them

If you have cracking, rough fingernails, it can look like you've been digging ditches all day—with your hands.

Women can use nail polish to try and cover the problem up…and lots of guys will just ignore the issue.

But that can be a big mistake—because your fingernails can actually be a quick indicator of your health and a potentially serious vitamin shortage. And getting your vitamin levels up to snuff can be an easy way to improve your fingernail health and even ward off disease!

Believe it or not, just looking at your fingernails can tell you if you're suffering from a significant vitamin B12 deficiency.

Vitamin B12 is actually crucial to fingernail health. And when you don't have enough, you can notice heavy ridges on your nails and that white "crescent moon" at the nail base disappearing.

Now, of course, a B12 deficiency can come with plenty of other symptoms, like fatigue and mental fog that you may have noticed. And maybe you've even gotten a B12 shot over the years to help improve your energy levels.

But what many people don't know is that we have a much tougher time absorbing B12 as we get older. So lots of seniors in particular end up deficient.

You can try taking large doses to make sure your body absorbs some of it. But your best bet is probably to get tested and then get B12 injections.

By injecting the B12 right into your muscles, you bypass your digestive system that might not be able to properly absorb the nutrient.

And loading up on B12 won't just make your fingernails look good again. You also may get the upper hand on more serious disease.

In fact, studies have shown that being low on B12 can make you a sitting duck for depression and cognitive decline, including symptoms that can mimic dementia and Alzheimer's.

So taking B12 isn't just about improving your fingernails—it may even improve your quality of life.

Get Supermodel Skin With These Oil Tricks

You can work out, eat well, and try just about everything under the sun to look younger.

But nothing makes you look older than wrinkles, rough skin, and skin blemishes.

Luckily, there are easy ways to take care of your skin without spending a fortune with a dermatologist. By using the right oils, you can effectively treat skin conditions like acne, eczema, calluses, scarring and even sunburn.

Here are the five best essential oils for giving you youthful, beautiful skin:

Skin Secret #1: Tea tree oil

The antibacterial and anti-fungal properties in tea tree oil effectively fight acne-causing bacteria and reduce inflammation and redness.

The best way to banish acne with tea tree oil is by applying it undiluted, with a cotton-tipped applicator, directly to the acne spots on your face.

For more severe acne, you can mix 6 drops of tea tree oil

with 3 tablespoons of witch hazel and spritz it on your face (not your eyes) once throughout the day.

Skin Secret #2: Lavender oil

Lavender oil has antibacterial, antiseptic, anti-fungal, moisturizing, calming and anti-inflammatory properties. It increases the speed of skin healing and reduces the appearance of scarring.

Because of this, it is one of the best oils used by alternative doctors for treating mild breakouts or eczema. It can be applied undiluted directly to your skin a few times each day until the spots or blotchiness are completely healed.

It can also be used as a preventative by mixing it with your favorite facial moisturizer.

Skin Secret #3: Myrrh oil

Myrrh is one of those cures that comes straight from the Bible (remember, it was one of the gifts given to the baby Jesus).

It has a wide array of benefits but is particularly helpful for skin that is scarred or aging. It has anti-inflammatory properties that brighten your skin tone, increase firmness and improve skin elasticity, which can dramatically reduce the appearance of wrinkles and scars.

Myrrh oil has a distinct smell that some people may not like, so it is probably best to use it at night, before you go to bed. Simply add a single drop into your normal moisturizer and apply directly to your face.

Skin Secret #4: Oregano oil

Oregano oil has strong antiviral, antibacterial and anti-fungal properties which make it the go-to oil for treating stubborn calluses on your feet.

You can treat calluses by adding a drop or two of oregano

oil with coconut oil and massaging the mixture directly onto your feet at night. After you rub the oil in, cover your feet with socks and leave them on until the next morning. After just a few days, you should notice a drastic reduction of the thick and uncomfortable calluses on your feet.

Skin Secret #5: Chamomile oil

If you are sensitive to the sun at all, even sunscreen can't save you from an occasional sunburn. Fortunately, you can drastically reduce the pain and appearance of sunburn using chamomile oil.

Chamomile is a mild, non-drying oil that can be applied directly to your skin, but for a particularly bad sunburn it is recommended that you mix 10 drops of chamomile oil with approximately 4 teaspoons of aloe vera and apply directly to the burned area of skin.

Many people are concerned that adding oil to their skin could cause clogged pores or other adverse reactions. However, the anti-fungal and antibacterial properties that are found in many essential oils prevent these problems.

A good supplier of essential oils is Piping Rock at **www.pipingrock.com.**

STOP Vision Problems with These 5 Underground Treatments

For years you've been told that vision loss is just a normal part of aging.

Go to your doctor with the problem, and he'll just sigh and recommend stronger glasses—or, if the problem is serious enough, even surgery.

But what you won't hear is that there are all-natural remedies that can help protect your eyes, no matter your age.

That's because many natural, herbal treatments are rich in antioxidant and immune-boosting phytochemicals that can ward off free radical damage that can do a number on your eyes.

Herbs and other kinds of plants have been used in healing for centuries, including for eye problems. Here are 5 of the best natural sight-savers around.

Sight-Saver #1: Bilberry

A relative of the strawberry and blackberry plants, bilberry has the same high concentration of vitamin C and other antioxidants.

Bilberry extract is often added to vitamin supplements for

treating eye problems, and it can also help support good night vision. Bilberry extract is available in capsule form and may also be added to herbal tea preparations.

Puritan's Pride makes a 1,000 mg. bilberry extract you can buy at **www.puritan.com**.

Sight-Saver #2: Black currant

Black currant has the same protective effects on the eyes as bilberry. Taken in capsule form as an extract or brewed as tea, black currant supports healthy circulation and increases blood flow to the eyes.

It also helps eyes adapt quickly to darkness and aids night vision. The antioxidants in black currant can also prevent eye damage from sunlight. You can pick up black currant supplements at **www.iherb.com**.

Sight-Saver #3: Gingko biloba

Long a staple of herbal healing in many cultures around the world, gingko biloba supports healthy circulation and increases blood flow throughout the body.

For that reason, it can encourage blood flow to the retina and may slow vision problems. Gingko biloba is also rich in antioxidants, which can protect the eyes from the damaging effects of UV radiation in sunlight.

This popular herb is available as an extract in capsule form, or as an herbal tea, and you can get supplements at **www.iherb.com.**

Sight-Saver #4: Green tea

Green tea's health benefits are well known, and the same properties that make it an immune boosting powerhouse for general good health can also support vision. The catechins and antioxidants in green tea help protect against free radicals and damage from UV exposure, and encourage blood flow to the retina and other tissues.

You can buy green tea as a supplement or pick up some for brewing at just about any supermarket.

Sight-Saver #5: Saffron

An essential nutrient for eye health is beta-carotene, found not only in orange and yellow vegetables and fruits, but also in brightly colored saffron. Saffron is a spice rich in carotenoids and phytochemicals that protect the eyes from damage caused by free radicals and UV light.

You can buy saffron supplements from Piping Rock at **www.pipingrock.com.**

How to Remove Warts WITHOUT Going to the Doctor

Warts can be ugly and disfiguring. But to get them removed, most people either have a doctor freeze them off or try those drug store remedies that are loaded with heavy-duty chemicals.

But there are natural wart treatments that are sitting in your home right now. They may take some time to work, but they're safe, cheap, and get good results.

One of the simplest natural methods is to apply pineapple juice to the wart with a piece of tissue or a cotton bud. The active ingredient is a mild form of acetic acid that literally eats away at the affected tissue, which is then slowly replaced by healthy skin.

While the process may sound a bit drastic, it is perfectly safe if done properly. You can easily apply the juice in the evening while you watch TV, and then allow it to dry when you go to bed. Repeat the procedure each day until the wart fades away.

You also can use a small fragment of pineapple under a breathable band-aid. Just apply it every night before you go to bed and then remove it in the morning to allow the skin to recover during the day.

A piece of fresh garlic clove can also be used under a band-aid, as long as you don't mind the mild odor that accompanies this remedy. Peel away the skin of the clove to uncover the juicy part of the garlic.

As with the pineapple fragment, cut away a small piece of fleshy garlic and apply it to skin, holding it in place with a band-aid or a piece of soft, breathable cloth. Note that there may some mild stinging with this remedy.

Unless this sensation becomes unbearable, it is worth continuing the treatment.

The third natural home remedy is to mix a small quantity of paste made from good quality honey and flaxseed, and apply this to the wart. A mortar and pestle is probably the best way to break the flaxseed open and effectively mix the two ingredients.

As you will need to apply the paste regularly over a number of days, it is a good idea to make a small quantity and keep it in an airtight jar until you need it.

Make sure that the consistency of the paste is such that it can be spread easily across the skin, but is thick enough to stay in place without creating a runny mess.

Once again, the paste should be held in place with a small, breathable bandage. Users report that this method is less painful than the pineapple and garlic, probably because the active ingredients are not acidic.

The main key with applying these methods is consistency. It will probably take a few days and sometimes even weeks to remove particularly large and troublesome warts, but the results will be worth it.

Hidden Natural Breakthroughs Kill Foot Fungus DEAD

If you've ever had toenail fungus, you know all about the ugly symptoms: peeling skin, irritation around the toes, and sometimes even pain and bleeding.

And if you've ever tried to treat the fungus, you know how stubborn it can be.

Fungal infections of the skin are generally caused by the tinea fungus, and can also appear on fingernails, around the genitals, and under folds of skin in obese people.

They are often worse in warm and humid weather (ideal growing conditions for fungus), and can keep coming back, even after you treat them.

The good news is that there are some natural breakthroughs that are proven effective against foot fungus. Just don't expect to learn about them in those Big Pharma fungus adds that run around the clock.

Fungus Remedy #1: Tea tree oil

Perhaps the best known of all remedies for tinea, tea tree oil is an anti-fungal that has earned its reputation. Dab a little onto the affected area several times a day, and you should see an improvement within a few days. Piping Rock is a good source for healing oils, at **www.pipingrock.com**.

Fungus Remedy #2: Wild oregano oil

This is a remedy that packs a punch in the world of fungus. Mix equal parts olive oil and wild oregano oil, and apply sparingly to the affected areas. Be sure you buy pure wild oregano oil with no alcohol or other additives.

Standard oregano oil is different and you won't get the results.

Fungus Remedy #3: Plain yogurt

Apply as a paste, and cover with a sock or glove. Leave for 30 minutes, then rinse off and pat dry.

Fungus Remedy #4: Apple cider vinegar

Dilute with equal amounts of water, and apply to the affected area several times a day. Leave to dry. You can also soak the infected area in the solution for 30 minutes, then pat dry. Continue doing this until the infection has cleared.

Fungus Remedy #5: Coconut oil

Is there anything coconut oil can't do? Coconut oil has excellent anti-fungal properties and is very mild. Simply rub it onto the affected area several times a day until the infection has cleared.

Fungus Remedy #6: Olive leaf

Olive leaf has great anti-fungal properties—take two spoonfuls of a tincture a day, or you can make a tea out of the dried leaves and drink two cups a day.

You can buy olive leaf tea at **www.teahaven.com.**

You don't have to put up with toenail fungus for the rest of your life. Using natural remedies like these, you can send toenail fungus packing!

This Oil Heals Stubborn Wounds ...So Why Isn't Anybody Talking About It?

When you think of ozone, you probably think of that big hole we have in the atmosphere…or the fresh smell after rainfall.

However, ozone also may hold the key to healing hard-to-treat wounds and other skin conditions.

Ozonated oils have been around since the early 1900s, but many people don't know about them and the mainstream isn't lifting a finger to promote them. One of these oils, ozonated olive oil, is practically a miracle for treating skin issues.

Ozonated olive oil is manufactured by inserting ozone (three oxygen atoms) gas into pure, unfiltered extra virgin olive oil.

As the gas bubbles through the oil, it develops a gel-like consistency that can be used as a healing, oxygen-rich salve on skin.

As with many popular health treatments, some manufacturers have started developing ozonated oil using processes that destroy its health benefits. When purchasing the oil, read the product label carefully to ensure that it is processed using a cold plasma oil generator.

Ozonated olive oil comes in both gel and liquid forms. The gel form contains 50 percent ozone, while the liquid form contains only 10 percent ozone. The gel version is slightly more beneficial than the liquid, because it absorbs more slowly and releases the healing effects over the course of 12 hours.

Ozonated olive oil has antibacterial properties that make it an effective treatment for cuts, wounds and skin conditions that are caused by bacteria, parasites or viruses. Unlike many oral antibiotics, you don't develop immunity to ozonated oil over time, so its effectiveness does not decrease.

You can also apply it as often as needed throughout the course of the day without fear of harmful effects. This oil also benefits those suffering from bacterial infections, such as ring worm and athlete's foot.

As a skin treatment, ozonated olive oil both disinfects and promotes faster healing in a variety of ailments. Some of the conditions that respond well to ozonated oil are sunburns, insect bites, hemorrhoids, diaper rash and dermatitis.

In addition to treating specific skin ailments, ozonated olive oil is an effective massage oil that draws toxins and excess lactic acid out of the skin.

As a wound healer and antibiotic, the oil also has many oral benefits and is used by dentists who combine alternative and conventional healing practices. Applying it to the gums and teeth after brushing can prevent or heal gingivitis and tooth decay. It is also a beneficial treatment for cold sores, ulcers and even severely chapped lips.

So what's the best way to get your hands on ozonated olive oil? You can buy a jar of purO3 at **www.honeycolony.com**.

Live 20 Years Longer with This Sacred Japanese Leaf

On the remote Japanese island of Hachijo, the residents have a secret that is stunning health researchers.

The island's inhabitants are regularly living into their 90s or even 100s.

They're energetic. Their minds are sharp. And they are regularly avoiding many of the deadly diseases that are killing off millions of seniors in other parts of the world.

So what's their secret?

Experts believe it's the sacred ashitaba plant...a longevity-promoting miracle that's been given the nickname the "Tomorrow Leaf."

Hachijo residents consume a lot of ashitaba in their diets, and its health secrets are the stuff of legend. It's believed to be the fabled "Elixir of Life" once sought by the first emperor of the Chinese Qin Dynasty, and thought to grant immortality to those who ate it.

The Tomorrow Leaf got its nickname from the plant's amazing ability to regrow plucked leaves within a day. That got health researchers wondering where its same restorative powers could be used to help people live longer, healthier lives.

It turns out that ashitaba is loaded with disease-fighting vitamins A, B, B2, B12, C, calcium, carotene, iron, fiber, potassium, and phosphorus.

And that's not all. It also contains a powerful antioxidant called chalcones.

Chalcones have been studied as preventatives for cancer, heart disease, hypertension, Alzheimer's, brain diseases, diabetes, osteoporosis, and mental fatigue.

In fact, in a 2014 study out of the University of California, Irvine, researchers found that chalcones may actually be able to target cancer at the cellular level.

"Compared to current cancer targeted therapeutic drugs, chalcones have the advantages of being inexpensive, easily available and less toxic," the researchers wrote.

A cheap, safe, and natural cancer fighter that you can literally pluck out of the ground? Don't expect to hear about that from the drug companies.

The people of Hachijo are living proof of ashitaba's age- and disease-fighting benefits. And there are lots of ways to incorporate it into your diet or supplement regimen.

In Japan, many people enjoy boiling the plant and eating it as a green. It's also eaten raw as a snack or in salads, and as a topping for noodles, casseroles, desserts, and other dishes in its powdered herbal form.

A good way to get ashitaba's benefits is to drink it as a tea. The leaves are first boiled, then slowly steeped to harness the plant's valuable nutrients.

Since the plant has a characteristic bitter taste, when it consuming as a tea, it's best to sweeten it with honey or other sweeteners.

If you want to give ashitaba a try, you can buy Percent Ashitaba Tea at **www.iherb.com.**

You can also buy Full Spectrum Japanese Ashitaba from Swanson Health Products at **www.swansonvitamins.com.**

Give Yourself a Natural HGH Boost—*Without* the Needles

It's the "stay young" secret of the Hollywood elite—including those leading men and starlets who always seem to look 10 or 20 years younger than they are.

Sylvester Stallone has used it for years to keep looking like Rocky, even as the years piled up.

It's human growth hormone—and if you're looking to keep muscle, shed fat, and stay mentally alert, HGH is the secret you've been looking for.

Unfortunately, HGH has gotten a notorious reputation over the years, thanks to abuse by professional athletes looking to hit more homeruns or sack more quarterbacks. And even the synthetic HGH injections offered by doctors can come with serious, nasty side effects.

But the good news is that there are some easy ways to give yourself a natural HGH boost and feel younger—without going near a needle.

We'll share the secrets in a minute. But first let's take a minute to understand what HGH does, and why it's so crucial to helping you look and feel young.

HGH is a hormone secreted by your pituitary gland, and it's essential for growing and repairing your cells.

But here's the problem—your HGH production peaks when you're young, and by the time you hit your 60s, you may only be producing and releasing about 20 percent of what you once were.

Replenishing your HGH levels can have real and lasting benefits for your health, including:

- Increased energy
- Improved immune system
- Growth of lean muscle tissue
- Increased bone density
- A better mood
- Improved fat burning abilities
- Younger looking skin
- A healthier sex drive

So how do you boost your HGH levels? Well, you can follow the lead of lots of sports stars and get injections. But the synthetic hormones many doctors use come with nasty side effects, including swelling of the limbs, carpal tunnel syndrome, and even the growth of "man boobs."

Who wants that? Some research even suggests that the long-term use of synthetic HGH injections can increase the likelihood of diabetes and cancer.

Fortunately, you don't have to turn to synthetic injections to give your body the HGH boost it needs. There are plenty of supplements on the market that can actually jumpstart your HGH production naturally, without the side effects.

Supplements that are designed to boost HGH production usually contain one or more ingredients that are capable of giving the pituitary gland the stimulation it needs to increase its hormone production rate.

Some options also contain ingredients that have been added to promote better sleep. This is important because the pituitary gland produces most of its HGH while the body is sleeping.

A few popular supplements proven to boost HGH include:

L-arginine: Studies have shown that this amino acid actually increases how much HGH your pituitary gland releases. Most of the research has involved doses of 5–9g. When you exercise along with taking L-arginine, it can magnify the effect, according to a study out of Syracuse University.

NOW Foods makes an L-arginine supplement and you can find a local retailer at **www.nowfoods.com**.

GABA: GABA is a neurotransmitter that is often used in sleep formulations. But it's also a powerful HGH booster. A study out of Italy more than 20 years ago found that GABA can significantly increase HGH levels in your body. And by promoting sleep, GABA can help with HGH production as well.

You can pick up GABA from Puritan's Pride at **www.puritan.com.**

L-Glutamine: This is an essential amino acid for synthesizing protein, and it can also quickly elevate HGH levels. In a study published in the *American Journal of Clinical Nutrition*, people who took L-Glutamine saw increases in circulating HGH in less than an hour!

Check out **www.nowfoods.com** to see where you can pick up their L-Glutamine supplement near you.

Magnesium and zinc are also known to be effective HGH boosters, but both are easily lost from the body. So if you take them, make sure you're combining them with vitamin B6, which helps magnesium and zinc stay in the body longer.

CHAPTER 7:

ERASE NAGGING PAIN *WITHOUT* DRUGS OR SURGERY

Let This Calming Mineral Soothe Away Even the Worst Pain

If you're living with pain, you know the search for relief is practically non-stop.

You've popped all the dangerous and addictive pills. You've tried the creams and balms that leave you smelling like a candy cane all day.

Maybe you've even had some doctor tell you that you need to go under the knife for some risky surgery.

But soothing and relaxing away the worst joint and muscle pain doesn't have to be so difficult or expensive. Because scientists have now proven that...

The TRUE secret to pain relief is one of the simplest (and safest) minerals around!

It's magnesium, and it's been used for ages to help improve heart health, calm stress and soothe jittery nerves. But now we know that magnesium also holds the key to banishing pain—and keeping it away for good.

You see, when you're experiencing pain, your body starts pumping out excess levels of a neurotransmitter called N-Methyl-D-aspartic acid (NMDA) that relays pain messages to your brain.

There are actually prescription pain medications that are sold to block the action of NMDA—but magnesium can have the same effects, but without the risks that come with these drugs.

That means real—and *lasting*—pain relief without drugs.

In one study, 80 people with lower back pain were asked to take either a placebo or a magnesium supplement.

The patients who took magnesium **decreased their pain nearly 40 percent**—and, even better, they were still experiencing pain relief when researchers followed up with them 6 months later.

Just imagine—what would that kind of pain relief mean for you and your quality of life?

And magnesium doesn't just work for muscle and joint pain. In fact, how does this sound…

42% fewer migraines in just weeks!

In a landmark study published by the International Headache Society, 81 patients with migraines took either 600 mg. of magnesium or a placebo daily for 12 weeks.

These people were suffering an average of nearly 4 migraines a month…those painful, nauseating episodes that can leave you curled up in a dark room for hours on end.

But that's before magnesium went to work. The patients who took magnesium experienced nearly 42 percent fewer migraines in just 12 weeks!

That's the kind of real (and safe) relief that migraine sufferers have been hunting for years!

Magnesium is simply one of the most powerful pain relievers around. In fact, magnesium is so effective at stopping pain that it's even been used to help patients feel better faster after major surgery!

In one study, women who were undergoing hysterectomies were given doses of magnesium before their operations. These women experienced so much less pain after their operations that they were even able to cut back on the amount of morphine they used! That's right...

Less morphine (and pain) after MAJOR surgery, thanks to this miracle mineral!

With results like these, you'd think our government and mainstream doctors everywhere would be recommending magnesium to all of their patients.

But the fact is, the billion-dollar drug companies would never let that happen.

Pain medication is big business for the drug companies, and that business is booming.

The pain drug market is now worth about $30 billion a year—and with America's population aging, the sky is the limit.

Big Pharma—and their government lapdogs—have a vested interest in making sure you never know about natural pain relievers like magnesium.

Now the good news is that magnesium is a natural mineral, and you can get it from magnesium-rich foods like dark, leafy greens, whole grains, nuts, seeds, and even fish.

But if you think you're getting enough magnesium in your diet, you may be in for a BIG surprise. That's because lots of the processed foods we eat today are literally having the magnesium stolen right from them!

When vegetables and grains are processed today, they're actually separated into components that remove much of the magnesium content.

Some vegetables now have as much as 80 percent less

magnesium than they did before the 1950s, and the processing of grains and pasta can remove 80-95 percent of total magnesium.

That's right—as you get older and need magnesium MORE, you're actually getting less and less of it from your food.

It's no wonder that research shows that three-fourths of Americans aren't getting enough magnesium in their diets!

The best way to make sure you're getting the magnesium you need to control your pain is by supplementing. Look for magnesium citrate, which is absorbed best by your body.

You can buy magnesium citrate supplements at **www.pureformulas.com.**

Another interesting fact about magnesium is that it can be absorbed through the skin. So taking Epsom salt baths is another easy way to boost your magnesium levels.

That's an old pain-relief trick that mom probably recommended to you decades ago—and now we know it works.

The "Devil's Secret" to Banishing Back Pain

If you suffer from chronic back pain, you know how quickly it can wreck your quality of life.

It hurts to stand. It hurts to sit. And getting a good night's sleep…without tossing and turning…is nearly impossible.

Back pain is actually one of the leading reasons Americans miss work. And, unfortunately, it's also a top reason that people end up addicted to powerful (and potentially dangerous) prescription painkillers.

But imagine if you could get an upper hand on your back pain in just a few short weeks. Imagine being able to hit the golf links or work in your garden without worrying about those sudden, sharp spasms of pain.

It's all possible, thanks to a weird plant that you probably wouldn't think about touching…let alone eating.

This miracle pain soother is called devil's claw, and it grows in Southern Africa in places like Botswana and Namibia. And it gets it's scary sounding name because it's covered with small, sharp hooks.

But African healers have been using devil's claw for centuries to treat everything from fevers to kidney problems. And now we know that devil's claw is loaded with powerful, inflammation-fighting compounds called glycoside and harpagoside that can send back pain packing in just weeks.

In one study out of Germany, published in the *European Journal of Anaesthesiology*, nearly 200 men with back pain were assigned to take either a placebo or a devil's claw extract for 4 weeks.

And the men who took devil's claw were up to three times more likely to end up pain-free for five days in a row than the guys taking placebo.

Ask yourself—when was the last time you had five pain-free days?

And in another study that lasted more than a year, patients with back pain who took devil's claw experienced just as much pain relief as those taking the prescription drug Vioxx.

And you can bet that devil's claw was a lot safer, too. Remember, this is the same Vioxx that was later pulled off the market after a string of heart attacks.

Better still, devil's claw seems to be effective for lots of different types of pain. In a study published in *Phytomedicine*, the majority of people with back, knee or hip pain who took devil's claw reported less pain and more mobility in just 8 weeks.

The dose used in that study was 60 mg. daily.

As a supplement, devil's claw is becoming much more widely available. You can buy Nature's Way Standardized Devil's Claw Extract at **www.luckyvitamin.com.**

The Indian Chef's Trick for Smooth, Comfortable Joints

It's a mystery that's been puzzling health researchers for years... you might even call it the "Indian Paradox."

India's population has swelled to more than a billion people—about three times the size of the United States. But India only has about HALF as many people living with the constant pain of osteoarthritis.

So what's the secret? Well, don't ask Indian doctors—you'd be better off asking Indian chefs instead.

Because there's a common kitchen spice that India's people eat by the ton—and it may hold the secret to giving you the comfortable, pain-free joints you deserve.

It's turmeric, that spice that gives curry its bright yellow color. But now researchers say that turmeric is packed with a powerful inflammation-fighter called curcumin that goes to work fast to soothe achy joints.

You see, inflammation may be the single greatest threat to the health of your joints. It's what leaves them feeling so stuff, uncomfortable and inflexible all the time.

But curcumin actually blocks your body's natural COX-2

pathway that causes inflammation (that's the same pathway that's targeted by heavy-duty prescription drugs).

Curcumin is also a powerful antioxidant that can help prevent oxidative damage to your joints and just about everywhere else on your body.

And the research behind curcumin and joint health is nothing short of jaw-dropping.

In one lab animal study out of Canada, researchers found that curcumin actually blocks the activity of an enzyme that breaks down the collagen in your joints (a major risk factor for joint problems).

And in a 2012 study out of Baylor University, researchers gave patients with rheumatoid arthritis either 500 mg. a day or curcumin, diclofenac sodium (a common pain drug) or a combination of the two.

It turned out these patients didn't need drugs at all!

In fact, the folks taking curcumin alone had the best improvements in their Disease Activity Score (a measure of the severity of their condition) and the American College of Rheumatology's scale for joint swelling and tenderness.

In other words, curcumin ran circles around this prescription drug that's being handed out to countless people with joint pain every single day.

So how do you put the power of curcumin to work for you? Well, adding more turmeric to your diet it an easy way to start.

But your best bet is to take a concentrated curcumin supplement. One product worth trying is Doctor's Best Curcumin C3 Complex, which you can buy at **www.jet.com**.

Ease Fibromyalgia with This Baltimore Doctor's Cocktail

Living with fibromyalgia can leave you feeling like you were run over by a truck...every single day.

Your muscles and joints are so sore and tender that even the slightest touch can deliver waves of agony. And you can spend your days feeling exhausted and depressed.

And the worst part about fibromyalgia is that for years the mainstream medical establishment denied it was a legitimate condition at all. Countless patients were told that their symptoms were all in their heads, or that there was nothing wrong with them.

In fact, alternative doctors were the only physicians who took fibromyalgia seriously.

One alternative doctor even set out to develop a powerful remedy that some patients say has relieved even their worst fibromyalgia symptoms.

And you may feel a big difference after just a few treatments.

This fibromyalgia fighter is called the Myers cocktail, and it's a vitamin infusion that contains a combination of B vitamins, vitamin C, dexpanthenol, calcium, adrenal cortical extract, glycerin, magnesium, and glutathione.

Many fibromyalgia sufferers swear by this cocktail and claim that it provides more relief than anything else they've tried.

The Myers cocktail was developed by Dr. John Myers, a physician from Baltimore, who pioneered intravenous (IV) vitamins and minerals as part of treatment protocols for different medical conditions. And more doctors are wondering whether fibromyalgia may be triggered by deficiencies in key nutrients, like magnesium or B vitamins.

After Myers' death in 1984, Dr. Alan Gaby began treating many of his patients with the Myers cocktail and documenting his results.

And the results have been astounding!

In case studies published by Gaby in *Alternative Medicine Review*, the Myers cocktail delivered impressive results for fibromyalgia sufferers incredibly fast.

In one case, a 48-year-old woman claimed her symptoms had vanished after the first treatment! But even Gaby admits that's unusual—the patients who have experienced significant benefits, he claims, usually needed 3–4 treatments.

Myers and Gaby believed the key to reducing symptoms was to deliver nutrients intravenously, so higher concentrations reach your bloodstream and your cells.

The Myers cocktail is administered via an IV drip, which takes about 30 minutes, usually every few weeks for people with chronic conditions such as fibromyalgia.

While the Myers cocktail is still a bit of an underground remedy, more integrative physicians are starting to offer it. Go to the American College for Advancement in Medicine website at **www.acam.org** to find an integrative doctor near you, and call to see if he's offering the cocktail.

If he's not, there's a good chance he knows someone who is.

Can This Odd Jewelry Stop Migraine Nausea?

Anyone who thinks a migraine is just a headache has never had one.

Aside from pain, migraines come with their share of debilitating symptoms like sensitivity to light and nausea that makes even looking at food impossible.

But if you suffer from migraine nausea, you don't have to just "wait it out" any longer.

Breakthrough research from Dr. Zoltan Medgyessy, a leading German physician, has now shown that you can relieve migraine nausea naturally with just a small piece of jewelry.

An acupressure wristband, to be exact.

Dr. Medgyessy's study was conducted at the prestigious Berolina Clinic in Lohne, Germany.

Forty-one patients were asked to use acupressure wristbands during migraine attacks, and to complete an in-depth questionnaire after. In the three months before the study, the patients reported nausea intensity that averaged a 6.2 out of 10 on a common scale.

But that was before they started wearing acupressure

wristbands.

During the study, a staggering **83 percent of patients** noticed a reduction in their nausea. In fact, on average, their nausea intensity was cut in HALF in just 28 minutes flat!

Real nausea relief…a difference you can feel.. in less than half an hour? It's no wonder that 98 percent of patients said they'd be willing to use acupressure wristbands to prevent their migraine nausea.

The idea of acupressure to relieve nausea isn't exactly new. Acupressure has been used for ages to relieve stress, improve circulation, and release muscle tension in the body.

Even the famous Memorial Sloan Kettering Cancer Center offers instruction to chemotherapy patients on how to perform acupressure…and stimulate the body's trigger points…to reduce nausea.

The key pressure point targeted by acupressure bracelets (and the Memorial Sloan Kettering training) is known as P6, which is located on the inside of your wrist.

While you can learn to perform acupressure on yourself, bracelets that put pressure on P6 are easy to buy.

You can pick up Sea Band Nausea Relief Acupressure wristbands at major online retailers, like **www.target.com** and **www.walmart.com**.

Heartbroken Dad Discovers Underground Joint Breakthrough!

As parents, we'd do anything for our kids. And there's nothing worse than watching a child you love suffering from constant pain...and knowing there's nothing you can do to help.

But that's the exact situation that Dr. Alan Moore found himself in more than 20 years ago. His daughter Anne Marie was suffering from rheumatoid arthritis—and her joints had gotten so bad, that by the time she was in her 20s, she was using an electric wheelchair.

Nothing that Dr. Moore or Anne Marie tried was working. But instead of getting mad, Dr. Moore got busy.

He worked tirelessly in his kitchen, trying to craft a new joint formulation to help his daughter.

And his hard work paid off—because we now have Dr. Moore to thank for one of the greatest joint-health breakthroughs in a generation. It's a powerful substance that finally gave Anne Marie the joint relief she'd spent years hoping for—and there's a good chance it can do the same for you.

This joint discovery is called undenatured type II collagen, or UC-II. And it's actually made from the collagen of everyday farm chickens.

As you probably know, collagen is an important building block for healthy joints. It gives your joints the cushioning they need so you can climbs the stairs, go for a walk, or even mow your lawn without every step causing you agony.

And UC-II goes straight to your joints to help rebuild this important cushioning and give you the comfortable, flexible knees, hips, fingers, and shoulders that you deserve.

In fact, in one 90-day international study, published in the *International Journal of Medical Science,* UC-II blew away glucosamine and chondroitin—two of the most popular joint supplements around.

At the end of the study, which looked at patients with knee arthritis, researchers analyzed patients' pain and mobility with common scales used by doctors everywhere.

And UC-II was consistently **2–3 *times more effective*** than a combination of glucosamine and chondroitin.

In fact, patients taking UC-II experienced a whopping 40 percent improvement on one common arthritis measure called the visual analog scale.

And that was after just 90 days!

"UC-II treated subjects showed significant enhancement in daily activities suggesting an improvement in their quality of life," the authors wrote.

And that's really what it's all about, right?

In another study, patients who experienced knee pain after working out took 40 mg. of UC-II for 120 days. And at the end of the study, they could extend their knees farther and exercise longer without pain.

Sounds good, right?

UC-II may be one of the newer joint-care breakthroughs on the market, but supplement suppliers are catching on to its wonders fast.

You can buy NOW Foods UC-II supplements at **www.iherb.com**.

4 Easy Home Remedies for Tension Headaches

Tension headaches can strike out of the blue and can put a real damper on your day.

And if you're like a lot of people, you don't want to sit around waiting (and hoping) for aspirin to work. Plus, over time aspirin can do significant damage to the lining of your gut.

Luckily, there are four easy remedies that can help relieve tension headaches—without resorting to drugs.

Headache-Buster #1: Peppermint oil

Gently massaging peppermint oil to key areas where tension is stored is a wonderful way to relieve a tension headache, especially if you enjoy the cooling sensation from the peppermint oil.

Apply the peppermint oil to your temples, forehead, and the back of your jaw. The temples and forehead are obvious places, but most people are unaware that tension in their jaws contributes to headaches as well. Many people clench their jaw or teeth when they are stressed or agitated.

For those who have sensitive skin, test the peppermint oil

on the back of your hand to determine whether or not it irritates your skin. If it does, try the test again after diluting the oil with water or olive oil.

Headache-Buster #2: Cayenne

Have you ever eaten something spicy and felt relief from a headache or another type of pain?

The reason some spicy food reduces pain is that some spices contain capsaicin, which inhibits Substance P in your body. Substance P is partly responsible for the feeling of pain.

Cayenne is a spice high in capsaican, so it serves as a great home remedy for alleviating tension headaches, and you probably have some sitting in your spice rack.

One effective remedy involves dabbing a cayenne and water mixture in your nose. Dilute ½ teaspoon of cayenne powder in ½ cup of warm water. Next, soak a cotton swab in the cayenne solution ensuring you stir it around.

Gently apply the soaked cotton swab inside one nostril and then the other until your headache has disappeared or diminished. You will feel a slight burning sensation when sticking the cayenne swab in your nostril, which is a sign it's working.

Headache-Buster #3: Apple cider vinegar

For many centuries, apple cider vinegar has been used as a remedy for just about everything. Apple cider vinegar can relieve tension headaches as well.

Boil three cups of water and then pour the boiling water into a large bowl of ¼ cup apple cider vinegar. Drape a towel over your head for the purpose of trapping the steam and hover your face over the bowl as close as you can without the steam burning your face.

Deeply inhale the steam for about 5–10 minutes. Drink a

glass of water when you're finished and your headache should be gone or feel much better.

Headache-Buster #4: Almonds

Eating one or two handfuls of almonds sometimes relieves a tension headache because they contain salicin, which is commonly added to painkillers. In fact, the main ingredient in white willow, which has a chemical structure similar to aspirin, is salicin.

Is This "Vine of the Gods" the Next Rheumatoid Arthritis Breakthrough?!?

When you're diagnosed with rheumatoid arthritis (RA), it's hard to know what's worse—the crippling, disfiguring joint pain, or the medications you're taking to prevent it.

Because RA is an autoimmune disease...one where your immune system actually attacks and damages your joints... many people are put on drugs that suppress their immune systems.

That can make you a sitting duck for dangerous infections and diseases, including tuberculosis!

But the Chinese claim they've been sitting on a natural remedy for RA for ages. Unfortunately if you live in the United States, it can be a little difficult to get your hands on it (we'll show you how in a moment).

Thunder god vine (tripterygium wilfordii) has been used in traditional Chinese medicine to treat inflammatory disorders like RA.

Believe it or not, thunder god vine is actually a poisonous plant, and only the interior of the root is not toxic. So it needs to be prepared in a special way by formulators who know what they're doing.

But thunder god vine is sold all across China right now as both a supplement and a cream for joint pain.

And it's delivered impressive results for people suffering from RA.

In a study conducted in China and reported in the *British Medical Journal's Annals of the Rheumatic Diseases*, 207 patients with RA were separated into three groups.

The first group received thunder god vine extract. The second group received methotrexate, a drug commonly prescribed for RA and sold under brand names like Trexall and Rasuvo.

The third group received a combination of both remedies.

When it came to controlling joint pain and inflammation, thunder god vine was actually more effective than the methotrexate that may be sitting in your medicine cabinet right now.

And that's good news, because methotrexate is a powerful drug that's also used for chemotherapy, and it comes with side effects like diarrhea, stomach pain, dizziness, and even convulsions!

If you're currently taking methotrexate, you may have experienced some of these side effects firsthand.

Even if you want to continue taking methotrexate, the study found that thunder god vine made the drug work better.

Thunder god vine is a true underground remedy, so getting your hands on it can be a little tricky. If you have a practitioner in traditional Chinese medicine in your market, he might be able to give you a reliable formulation.

You can also buy a 200 mg. supplement at **www.thundergodrootextract.com.**

The number of products on the market is fairly limited, but as we see more and more positive research on thunder god vine, expect that to change.

Stop Gout Flare-Ups with This Drug-Free Protocol

A gout flare-up can leave you feeling like you're constantly walking on razor blades. The pain can strike your knees, ankles, feet, and toes, and taking even a few steps can be torture.

You know that the problem is caused by the buildup of uric acid crystals in your joints. But lots of the medications on the market either don't work or seem to take forever.

You want (and deserve) fast relief. And now you can have it, thanks to this simple, safe...and completely drug-free... protocol.

The first step, of course, is diet. If you don't lower the levels of uric acid in your blood, you're never going to fully get your gout under control.

Luckily, there are foods you can eat that are proven to decrease uric acid. Just remember to consume more of these...

3 Proven Uric Acid Fighters

- Coffee (which is also great for inflammation)
- Cherries

- Foods rich in vitamin C, like oranges, grapefruits, and even red peppers.

And, naturally, there are some foods you'll want to avoid.

Specifically, you want to stay away from foods with purine, which gets broken down to uric acid in your body. Here are…

4 Foods You Should NEVER Eat with Gout

- Asparagus
- Sardines
- Mushrooms
- Scallops

Meat, fish, and poultry should be limited to less than four to six ounces per day, since these foods can cause a buildup of uric acid when you eat too much.

Next, you want to add proven gout-fighting supplements to your regimen. Two of the best are vitamin C and quercetin, a flavonol found in many different foods (especially red kidney beans).

Vitamin C is a powerful antioxidant and researchers have understood forever the important role it plays in healthy joints and managing pain. But it turns out it may make the difference in preventing gout and flare-ups.

A 20-year joint study published by Canadian and Harvard researchers found that men who consumed the most vitamin C (sometimes more than 1,500 mg. a day) had the lowest risk for gout.

The authors concluded that "supplemental vitamin C may be beneficial in the prevention of gout." And, aside from adding more vitamin C to your diet, vitamin C supplements are available at just about any supermarket or pharmacy.

Finally, quercetin is a proven inflammation-fighter, and controlling inflammation is critical to resolving joint issues.

A Chinese study published in 2012 gave quercetin to mice with gout, and the supplement reduced several of the key blood markers associated with inflammation. It also increased anti-oxidant activity, which is important to staving off joint damage.

Jarrow Formulas makes a 500 mg. quercetin supplement that you can buy at **www.allstarhealth.com**.

Fix Joint Woes with a Glass of "Super Water?"

Could soothing the constant pain and stiffness of rheumatoid arthritis (RA) be as simple as drinking a glass of water?

It could be—but only if you're drinking the right kind.

We know that RA is an autoimmune disease that attacks your joints and can lead to deformity and disability.

But science has proven time and time again that preventing oxidative stress—and controlling inflammation—are important to smoother, more comfortable joints.

So Japanese scientists decided to see whether drinking water with high concentrations of hydrogen, a powerful anti-oxidant, could provide relief for RA patients.

And the results were better than anyone could have expected.

The study had 20 RA-diagnosed participants drink half a liter of high-concentration hydrogen water for four weeks.

Next, they drank only hydrogen water, but at lower levels, for another four weeks. Lastly, the participants finished the study with four more weeks of high-concentration hydrogen water.

At the end of each four-week period, the participants were tested for blood indicators of RA and proteins that are related to disease activity.

All 20 participants experienced improvement in blood markers.

Sixteen of the 20 (that's 80 percent!) participants felt *major relief of RA symptoms.*

However, what was more incredible...nine of the participants experienced remission!

What would remission from your RA symptoms mean for you? Imagine being able to spend your days enjoying your favorite activities without the constant joint pain and stiffness.

Those are the results that real people...just like you... experienced with hydrogen water.

And while you may never have tried hydrogen water before, it's easy to start enjoying its health benefits right away.

You can pick up Active H Molecular Hydrogen Tablets from major online retailers, like **www.amazon.com**.

Or try searching "hydrogen water pitcher" online for filters that can make hydrogen-rich water straight from your tap water.

CHAPTER 8:

GET A YOUNGER BRAIN WITH THESE BLACKLISTED DISCOVERIES

Can This Strange Mushroom Actually REVERSE Dementia?!?

Being diagnosed with dementia—or even Alzheimer's disease—doesn't just steal your precious memories…or your personality…or your freedom to live independently and care for yourself.

Before the worst symptoms even set in, dementia can steal your sense of hope.

That's because you've been told that there's nothing you can do to fight it.

You've been told that mainstream medicine can't do anything to stop this dreaded disease from stealing nearly everything that makes you who you are.

And that's right—there's nothing that mainstream medicine can do.

But that's not the end of the story. Because clinical research has now shown that a powerful, underground remedy can actually help your brain heal itself. In fact, it's even been proven to…

Begin reversing dementia in *just 8 weeks!*

This dementia breakthrough is called lion's mane (*Hericium erinaceus*), and it's been used in traditional European and Asian healing for ages. It gets its name because it grows in strange long strands on tree bark.

And while it's not the kind of mushroom you're going to throw on top of a steak or into your dinner salad, it may hold the key to stopping (and reversing) memory loss.

In a double-blind, placebo-controlled study (the gold standard of research), 30 Japanese seniors with mild cognitive impairment were asked to take either 1,000 mg. of lion's mane a day or a placebo for 16 weeks.

And these seniors were living in very dangerous territory, because mild cognitive impairment is often the last step before full-blown dementia or Alzheimer's.

But the patients taking lion's mane actually began to reverse their memory loss and thinking problems, starting in just 8 short weeks.

They were measured using something called the Hasegawa Dementia Scale (HDS-R), which is one of the leading tools around for diagnosing dementia and memory problems.

And at the end of the 16-week study, the patients taking lion's mane had significantly improved their HDS-R scores.

That means they were actually *reversing* their symptoms of dementia!

But here's the best part—the improvements started in as little as 8 weeks! What would it be like to know that you may be able to think more clearly or remember better in just 8 short weeks?

And this isn't just a short-term fix either. In another clinical study on people with mild cognitive impairment and dementia, patients took Amyloban 3399 (a supplement extracted from lion's mane) for a year.

Patients with mild cognitive impairment or recent-onset dementia experienced dramatic improvements in their cognitive abilities. Amyloban 3399 even helped people who were experiencing brain problems as side effects of prescription medications, like antidepressants.

So how does lion's mane work? It actually targets your brain at the cellular level to turn back the clock on some of the damage we experience as we get older.

You see, our bodies produce a natural protein known as nerve growth factor, or NGF.

And NGF does exactly what it sounds like. It's responsible for the regulation and survival of the neurons in your brain. In fact, NGF actually determines which brain cells live—and which die.

But NGF comes with one big problem...

We have a healthy supply of NGF when we're younger. But our levels start to fall off as we age.

That can make us sitting ducks for serious brain problems—including dementia and Alzheimer's!

But that's what makes lion's mane so important. It actually stimulates natural production of NGF, helping precious brain cells survive—and thrive.

In one animal study, scientists proved that compounds from lion's mane can cross the blood-brain barrier, jumpstart NGF synthesis in the brain, and improve cognitive function.

And more NGF means a healthier brain— simple as that.

But believe it or not, increasing NGF production isn't the only way that lion's mane helps heal and protect your brain.

In a 2006 study out of Japan, published in the *Journal of Nutritional Biochemistry*, Amyloban from lion's mane actually protected brain cells from dying when they were exposed to beta amyloid peptides.

And if you've done some research on Alzheimer's, you know all about beta amyloid. The accumulation of sticky beta amyloid plaques in the brain is considered one of the leading causes of Alzheimer's disease.

According to the Alzheimer's Association, beta amyloid plaques actually interfere with communication among your brain cells. And they can even trigger inflammation and cause your immune system to attack and kill neurons!

Reducing beta amyloid in your brain is important to preventing memory loss and Alzheimer's disease. And lion's mane is a powerful way to fight back against these plaques.

So how do you get your hands on lion's mane? Well, it is edible—but it's not terribly popular in American cuisine.

Your best bet is to take lion's mane as a supplement. You'll find plenty of suppliers online, but you can actually buy the Amyloban 3399 that's been used in research studies.

You can purchase Mushroom Wisdom's Amyloban 3399 from Destination Vitamins at **www.destinationvitamins.com.**

It's sold in 180-capsule bottles, and you take two capsules three times a day. So 180 capsules should last you a full month.

Did Hurricane Katrina Uncover Secret Cause of Parkinson's?!?

If you or a loved one suffers from Parkinson's disease, it can feel like the bad news never stops coming.

The tremors, stiffness, fatigue, and mood changes can make life miserable—and you've been told they're only going to get worse.

For years the mainstream hasn't had a clue how to prevent Parkinson's or turn back some of the damage. But now it looks like we're on the cusp of a major breakthrough.

And, believe it or not, we may have Hurricane Katrina to thank.

I'm sure you remember Katrina like it was yesterday. When it struck in 2005, New Orleans and other towns along the Gulf Coast were practically destroyed.

More than 1,200 people died, and the property damages reached $108 billion.

But for Professor Joan Bennett, Hurricane Katrina was a major "eureka" moment.

You see, Bennett was working as a professor at Tulane University in New Orleans, and her home flooded. As the mold developed, she started developing serious neurological symptoms like constant headaches and dizziness.

And that's what got Bennett thinking—what other neurological problems might be caused by mold?

When she took a job at Rutgers University, she ended up teaming up with scientists from Emory University to study how mold may affect brain chemicals.

And that's when they made a pretty shocking discovery.

In a study on insects they learned that a common component in mold, 1-octen-3-ol (otherwise known as mushroom alcohol), has the power to kill off dopamine levels.

Dopamine is a key neurotransmitter, and declines in dopamine are a major trigger for Parkinson's and its symptoms.

In fact, Bennett and her colleagues now believe that mold may be what's causing a spike in Parkinson's cases in rural areas, where mold tends to be more prevalent.

The bad news is that there are many people who have been living with mold exposure for years. The good news is that there's something you can do about it.

You can find mold remediation specialists in your phone book, and they'd be happy to come to your home and charge a fortune for some mold tests.

But there's plenty you can do on your own before things get that far. There are home tests for mold that you can buy at places like Home Depot (or online) for less than $50.

The best place to start is by focusing on areas where water may have pooled—like around appliances, bathrooms, the insulation and flooring in your basement, or places where you had floods or leaks.

If you start to get some troubling results, it may be time for professional investigation and remediation (call your home insurer to see if any of it may be covered).

Mold removal can be costly. But we're learning that it may hold the key to preventing Parkinson's or keeping symptoms at bay.

Vitamin B12 For Your Brain? Throw it Out Until You Read *This!*

Do you ever get that "I know I should know this" feeling?

Or constantly have words at the tip of your tongue but can't ever seem to find them?

Then you may be one of the 16 million people in the U.S. suffering from a common condition called mild cognitive impairment, or MCI.

MCI is a precursor for dementia and is diagnosed when your brain functions are below what's normal from your age. When left untreated, MCI often results in full-blown dementia.

One reason MCI may happen to you is age-related brain shrinkage.

Fortunately, B vitamins, particularly vitamin B12, have been proven to slow down and even prevent memory decline and the brain shrinkage associated with age and MCI. This is especially true in folks who have elevated levels of homocysteine, a toxic chemical that encourages brain atrophy.

But now it looks like there's a whole lot more to the story.

Scientists have discovered that B vitamins are most potent against the negative effects of aging on the brain when taken with another vital nutrient.

In fact, an international research team has proven that without a healthy level of this powerful nutrient, B vitamins are rendered almost useless at shielding your brain from cognitive impairment.

For the study, 250 people who were afflicted with mild cognitive impairment were subjected to a battery of tests that measured their cognitive abilities. In addition, they also had a blood test that measured their levels of omega-3 fatty acids (commonly found in certain fish).

Then the volunteers were randomly split into two different groups, one of which took a B vitamin supplement and the other which took a placebo for the next two years.

And what they found was SHOCKING!

As it turns out, folks who had low levels of omega-3s saw almost no brain-protective benefits from taking the vitamin B supplements.

However, in folks who had high levels of omega-3s, the B vitamins "were very effective in preventing cognitive decline compared to the placebo."

This means if you're taking B vitamins, including B12, without taking omega-3s, you might was well be taking nothing at all.

Dr. Doug Brown, director of research and development at Alzheimer's Society, reports:

"These results help us to tease apart who could benefit from taking B vitamins, suggesting that they might only improve cognition in people who have high levels of omega-3 oils in their blood. Encouragingly, these findings suggest that for some older people a combination of fish oil supplements and B vitamins may help to improve thinking and memory."

Just imagine the number of seniors who are taking B vitamins for their brains right now, without realizing they're getting no benefit because their omega-3 levels are too low.

If you're currently taking B vitamins, be sure to couple them with a fish oil supplement.

But be cautious of which brand you choose. Only purchase fish oil supplements that have been molecularly distilled so they are free of contaminants.

You can pick up B-complex vitamins just about anywhere. But not all fish oil has been molecularly distilled.

A good source of molecularly distilled fish oil is Super Omega-3 from Wonder Laboratories. Just go to **www.wonderlabs.com.**

This Superstar's Secret Could *Save* You from Alzheimer's

Kris Kristofferson may be one of the most versatile performers of all time. From writing to singing to acting, he's literally done it all.

And while Kristofferson may have enjoyed a very uncommon career, when he reached his late 70s something *incredibly common* happened to him.

He was diagnosed with Alzheimer's he didn't have.

And, believe it or not, the same thing could happen to you or someone you love.

You see, one of the most closely guarded secrets in all of medicine today is that doctors' get Alzheimer's diagnoses wrong all the time.

Two studies published in 2016 examined the brains of thousands of patients who had been diagnosed with Alzheimer's before they died. Unfortunately, an autopsy is the only real way to confirm Alzheimer's.

But in 20 percent of those cases, the brain examinations revealed that the patients *never really had Alzheimer's at all.*

They spent the last years of their lives suffering from other, undiagnosed…and possibly treatable…conditions.

In fact, that's what almost happened to Kristofferson.

Once his memory started slipping, his doctors just assumed it was dementia.

He was the right age and had the symptoms, after all.

So they handed him some useless meds, sent him home, and basically told him life as he knew it was over.

And for years, he just kept getting worse.

But it wasn't Alzheimer's that was stealing Kristofferson's memory…*it was Lyme disease!*

You see, many people with Lyme disease are never properly diagnosed—and, when the disease is left untreated, it can mimic many of the symptoms of Alzheimer's.

Once an alternative doctor got the brilliant idea to test Kristofferson for Lyme…and once his Lyme was treated with antibiotics…the change was miraculous.

Within just a few weeks, his wife said, it was as if he'd come back to life. His memory improved and he was like his old self again.

"I'm just so grateful," she said.

The fact is, there are likely thousands of Americans right now who are in the same boat as Kristofferson. They've been wrongly diagnosed with Alzheimer's.

Never accept an Alzheimer's diagnosis for yourself or a loved one until you've received several opinions and have been tested for everything else that could cause your symptoms.

That can include Lyme disease, vitamin deficiencies, poor thyroid function, and even side effects from the drugs you're taking.

Slow Memory Loss to a Crawl with This Vitamin Fix

Whether it's forgetting where you left the keys, or mixing up your grandkids' names, those "senior moments" we get as we age are never fun.

Memory lapses aren't just an inconvenience—they can be downright frightening, especially as they get more frequent.

We've all gotten lots of advice over the years on how to keep our brains sharp. We read books, watch *Jeopardy*, and fill out the newspaper crossword puzzle every day.

But now scientists say protecting our precious memories may be as easy as popping a vitamin D supplement every day.

In a study published in the *Journal of the American Medical Association*, researchers from Rutgers University studied the memories and vitamin D levels for a group of seniors.

The seniors ranged from those with perfectly functioning memories to those with pretty serious dementia.

And those with dementia all seemed to have one thing in common—they were low in vitamin D.

People with the lowest vitamin D levels had more short-term memory loss and less ability to organize their thoughts and make decisions.

Their brains were actually declining a whopping *250% percent faster* than people with healthy vitamin D levels.

The fact is, vitamin D is essential to countless processes that occur within your body—including the normal functioning of your brain. Unfortunately, studies show that many people (especially seniors) are deficient in this vital nutrient.

Fortunately, there's something you can do about that. You can get vitamin D from some foods, like salmon, cheese, and egg yolks.

Your body also can make vitamin D naturally from the sun, which is why it's often called the "sunshine vitamin." So spending some time outside each day with your head and arms exposed can help.

Unfortunately, lots of our bodies get much less efficient at producing vitamin D as we age. And, depending on where you live, there may not be too much sunshine year-round.

That's why your best bet is to load up on vitamin D supplements. The Vitamin D Council and many physicians recommend a dose of around 2,000 IUs a day.

The most common form of vitamin D is D3 or cholecalciferol. This more closely matches the vitamin D produced naturally by your body.

[Warning] Popular Medical Test Could Damage Your Brain

Maybe you took a fall…or a blow to the head…or even suffered a stroke.

If so, there's a good chance that you've been sent for a CT scan.

Around 62 million Americans get these scans every year—and we've been told they're the only surefire way to see what's going on inside our heads.

But it looks like CT scans come with a hidden danger we've never been warned about.

An international research team has just discovered that CT scans can damage a part of your brain responsible for memory and learning.

That can put you on a path to Alzheimer's…and it can start with as little as one scan.

The big problem with CT scans won't come as much of a shock—it's the radiation.

There's more and more evidence showing that radiation exposure can lead to serious health issues—including damage to the hippocampus region of the brain

To investigate this further, the researchers exposed mice to chronic low doses of radiation 24 hours per day for a period for 300 days.

At the end of the experiment, the researchers examined the mice's brains…and what they found was mind-blowing!

The radiation didn't just damage the hippocampus; it actually changed it on a very basic level.

But what's more upsetting—these changes resemble features that are associated with Alzheimer's disease.

Unfortunately, the bad news doesn't end there.

The mice were exposed to only a tiny fraction of the amount of the radiation you would get from a CT scan.

In fact, the dosage given to the mice was so miniscule, it was over 1,000 times smaller than what most folks get during just one CT scan.

And even with this low of a dosage, the researchers still detected major changes in the parts of the hippocampus that are linked to Alzheimer's.

The only problem is CT scans aren't the only source of radiation you're exposed to. Things like flying on an airplane, going through security scanners and even some consumer products—like smoke detectors, certain TVs and eating produce that has been irradiated—can increase your radiation exposures.

We're surrounded by so much radiation—from medical imaging and other sources—that experts say our chances of developing Alzheimer's are set to skyrocket in the next decade.

Now, even many doctors admit that they use tests like X-rays and CT scans more than they probably need to. So any time a test is ordered, it's always a good idea to talk to your doc about whether it's necessary and what he's hoping to find.

And even though we can't eliminate medical imaging tests completely from our lives, there are some other simple ways to reduce our radiation exposure.

Opt for the pat down at the airport, turn off your television if you're not using it, and choose organic foods since they've not been irradiated.

There have also been some promising animal studies showing that the supplement N-acetyl cysteine (NAC) may help protect us from radiation damage. NAC basically helps your body maintain proper levels of glutathione, a powerful antioxidant that helps thwart cellular damage.

Because glutathione is so important to things like brain and heart health, it just makes sense to add NAC to your supplement regimen. Many alternative doctors recommend it religiously.

Pure Formulas makes NAC capsules you can buy at **www.pureformulas.com.**

Powerful Spice Fights Depression as Well as Prozac

The statistics on prescription antidepressants are, well…downright depressing.

Nearly 10 percent of Americans are now taking these meds, which come with serious side effects like weight gain, brain fog, loss of sex drive, and even suicidal thoughts.

With all of these problems, you'd think the mainstream would be more cautious about handing out antidepressants. But go to your doctor with a case of the blues, and you're practically guaranteed to leave with a prescription for Paxil, Prozac, Zoloft, or some other Big Pharma concoction.

Depression is a serious issue—but you don't need to put your health at risk to beat it.

In fact, there's a powerful natural solution that research proves is just as effective as Prozac. And it's a whole lot safer.

It's called curcumin.

It's the active ingredient in the spice turmeric and has been a key player in natural health for thousands of years.

More recently, it's been touted by health researchers for its anti-inflammatory and brain-protective properties in many studies.

And now it's proving to be a potent antidepressant.

A study published in the journal *Phytotherapy Research* involved 60 people diagnosed with major depressive disorder by a commonly used scale.

The first group took 20 mg of Prozac with 1g of curcumin. The second group took only 20mg of Prozac. The final group took 1g of curcumin alone.

At the end of the six-week trial, the patients were then given the assessment again.

What the researchers found next was astounding…

You see, once all the data were gathered, the scientists found that curcumin can fight depression just as well as Prozac!

"This study provides first clinical evidence that curcumin may be used as an effective and safe modality for treatment in patients with major depressive disorder," the authors wrote.

Curcumin is considered to be very safe in doses up to 12g a day. The participants in the study were getting only 1g—a tiny fraction of the possible daily dose of curcumin.

Just imagine how amazing the results might have been if they were given a larger dose!

Not to mention, curcumin has brain-protective powers, which may help improve your brain functions and ward off the age-related memory issues like dementia and Alzheimer's.

But here's the best part—unlike Prozac and other antidepressants, curcumin was well tolerated by all participants, which means they experienced little or no side effects. This is great news for folks who have suffered from the draining side effects of standard antidepressants.

This study has shown that curcumin is the all-natural breakthrough the antidepressant market needs.

If you're going to take curcumin supplements, be sure that the brand you select uses "optimized" or "free" curcumin. This type is easiest for your body to absorb and has the greatest impact on your health.

You can get optimized curcumin from the supplement supplier ProHealth at **www.prohealth.com**.

Ancient Tonic Could Keep You from Getting Parkinson's

Parkinson's disease is slow-developing, progressive neurological disease that slowly destroys your quality of life.

Most patients experience their first symptoms around the age of 60 or older, and they can be as benign as a barely noticeable tremor in the finger or hand.

Every year, over 60,000 Americans are diagnosed with Parkinson's disease.

But the numbers only start here.

Currently, there are as many 1 million Americans suffering from Parkinson's disease and an estimated 10 million people worldwide.

And these numbers don't include the thousands of cases that go undetected.

The best way to beat Parkinson's is to never get it in the first place.

Fortunately, there is a natural solution that can help reduce the risk of Parkinson's—one that has been used for centuries as a health booster.

So what is this Parkinson's fighter?

Yerba mate.

This South American plant is found in parts of Brazil, Paraguay, Argentina, and other South American countries. It's been used by the native peoples of these regions for both social and medicinal practices for centuries, typically as a tea.

However, a study released in the *Journal of the Neurological Sciences* reveals that yerba mate also has a protective role in the development of Parkinson's disease.

The study examined hospital records of those who drank yerba mate regularly. And it turns out that drinking yerba mate tea can reduce your risk of Parkinson's by a third!

Researchers believe yerba mate's bioactive compound content is one of the reasons why it's an effective Parkinson's preventative. These include xanthines, phenolics, theobromine, and caffeine.

Plus, yerba mate has more health benefits!

Yerba mate is full of natural phenolic compounds and antioxidants (natural cancer-fighters and metabolism boosters). It's also good for a quick pick-me-up, as it has a caffeine content equal to most coffees.

Not to mention yerba mate signals the body to burn more fat, regulates blood sugar levels, and helps reduce inflammation related to obesity.

While it can be enjoyed hot, the iced version can be refreshing treat as well.

This makes yerba mate a great choice for iced tea in the hot months of summer—you can quench your thirst while fighting Parkinson's and enjoying other health benefits!

Yerba mate is a leafy and at times even dusty loose tea. This can make for a gritty and cloudy iced tea experience.

Chemex brewing yerba mate is a great way enjoy it and to accentuate its refreshing and earthy flavor while also preventing leaves and other small particles from swimming in your glass.

You can pick up a chemex brewer at **www.chemexcoffee**

maker.com. You can also choose from several varieties of organic yerba mate tea and iced tea at **www.iherb.com**. You can easily buy a box for well under $10.

Weird Underwater Algae STOPS Memory Loss

Billion-dollar drug companies have spent a fortune trying to develop wonder pills that can stop or even reverse memory loss.

Get your hands on a bottle of these pills, and you've basically bought yourself an expensive paperweight—and nothing more.

Now it looks like these drug researchers should have stepped outside their labs and gone scuba diving instead. Because buried in the bottom of the ocean is a powerful algae that may hold the secret to preventing brain disease and keeping your mind young as you age.

It's called astaxanthin, and it's is a natural carotenoid (or pigment), found in microalgae. Astaxanthin is actually what gives algae their bright colors.

But that's not all it does. As a potent antioxidant and anti-inflammatory, astaxanthin is becoming the next big underground breakthrough for brain health and preventing memory loss.

You see, antioxidants like astaxanthin slow or prevent oxidative processes in the body that create damaging free radicals. And oxidative stress has been linked to many serious brain diseases, like Alzheimer's and Parkinson's.

So what makes astaxanthin so special? As a fat-soluble molecule, astaxanthin is one of the few nutrients able to cross the blood-brain barrier, sending its antioxidant and anti-inflammatory benefits straight to your brain tissue.

In a landmark double-blind, placebo-controlled study out of Japan (the same kind of study used on billion-dollar drugs) nearly 100 middle-aged people and seniors complaining of forgetfulness were asked to give astaxanthin a try.

After just 12 weeks, the folks taking astaxanthin showed amazing improvements on both cognitive function and learning tests. In fact, astaxanthin was shown to work at doses as low as 6mg. a day! The results were even better at 12mg.

Imagine that—better brain function in as little as three months!

And in another animal study, researchers actually discovered that astaxanthin works through an important molecular pathway that helps control your ability to remember things.

And, believe it or not, that's not all astaxanthin does. Studies have also found that astaxanthin improves production of certain neurotransmitters, improving memory and brain function.

Astaxanthin has also been shown to decrease a substance (phospholipid hydroperoxides) that accumulates in people suffering from dementia. It's like it actually shields your brain from this dangerous, memory-robbing substance.

So how do you get your hands on astaxanthin? You can pick up your own supply from Puritan's Pride at **www.puritan.com**.

They sell doses ranging from 4mg. to 10mg. The 10mg. dose is closer to what has been used in astaxanthin research.

Can Eliminating This ONE Food Prevent Alzheimer's?!?

Alzheimer's is the disease that many seniors fear the most as they age. It slowly robs you of your memories, your personality...even what it means to be you.

And this frightening disease is about to reach epidemic proportions. More than 5 million Americans are currently living with Alzheimer's, and that number is expected to triple in the next 25 to 30 years.

We keep hearing about all the research that's being done to treat Alzheimer's. But let's face it—mainstream drugs do practically nothing, and there are no promising medications on the horizon.

That's the bad news. The good news is that keeping yourself Alzheimer's-free may be as simple as making one simple dietary change.

You just need to cut processed foods out of your diet. This means those supermarket TV dinners and cookies, and whatever mystery food your local drive-through is serving.

You see, processed food contributes large quantities of

sugar to your diet. It is added to almost every manufactured food including bread, crackers, vegetables, canned fruits, complete meals, sauces, pizza, beverages, and many thousands of other items.

Even foods that do not taste sweet can contain lots of sugar. Processed foods in particular are loaded with excessive amounts of sugar while most contain no healthy fats.

And here's why that matters for your brain.

Researchers have discovered that the brain produces its own insulin that helps brain cells survive and thrive.

But when you consume too much sugar, especially the kinds found in processed foods, you develop a condition called insulin resistance where your cells can't use insulin properly.

Now you may know that insulin resistance is an early indicator of type 2 diabetes. But it also affects your brain cells and keeps them from working properly and surviving.

The connection between blood sugar and brain health has even led some researchers to call Alzheimer's disease "type 3 diabetes."

In 2013, the *New England Journal of Medicine* published a study proving that fasting blood glucose levels as low as 105–110 (which isn't even considered diabetic or pre-diabetic by some doctors) can send your risk of dementia through the roof.

If your blood sugar is in this range (or higher) it's essential to make serious dietary changes that start with eliminating processed foods.

In fact, did you know that just ONE SLICE of frozen pizza can add 6 grams or more of added sugar to your diet? And who eats just one slice anyway?

The best measure anyone can take to reduce their risk of developing Alzheimer's disease is to eat a healthy diet containing no processed foods. Every food can be made fresh at home, and it will taste better, be free of preservatives, and provide quality nutrients.

For easy ways to cut added sugars out of your diet—and for simple food substitutions, check out the "Eat This, Not That" website at **www.eatthis.com**.

Is Your iPhone Destroying Your Memory?

Let's face it—we don't go anywhere these days without our smartphones.

You can't even visit a restaurant or a golf course without seeing someone pulling out their iPhone or Android phone to check the latest news, texts from friends, and sports scores.

Nearly 70 percent of Americans own a smartphone. But they're not just a modern convenience—studies show they may be doing long-term damage to our memories and even how our brains operate.

Now some of that is just common sense. Research conducted by Kaspersky Lab has found that smartphones are basically making our brains lazy and under-utilized.

With so much information at our fingertips, smartphones keep us from having to remember when the Civil War ended, the lyrics from our favorite songs, or even our friends and family members' phone numbers.

In fact, the Kaspersky Lab study found that 71 percent of people can't recall their children's phone numbers, and nearly half couldn't remember their childhood phone numbers. Those statistics would have been unthinkable a generation ago!

Our memories are in free-fall!

Your brain is like a muscle—it needs exercise and practice remembering things, but smartphones are preventing it. Kaspersky Lab calls this "digital amnesia," as the brain gets sloppy at having to rely on itself for keeping tabs on what's going on in your world.

And more and more research is pointing to the long-term brain and memory changes from smartphones.

A study out of the Mayo Clinic discovered that texting produces a new type of brain rhythm that researchers had never even seen before!

And research from the Boston University School of Medicine even found that using smartphones and tablets may stunt kids' development of social and emotional skills. Look at a lot of the poorly-adjusted teenagers today, and you have all the evidence you need there.

Even worse, the effects of the blue light from phones on people's sleep is well documented. And research shows that when you don't get enough sleep, you're a sitting duck for cognitive decline.

With an estimated 71 percent of American smartphone users admitting to taking them to bed, chances are a lot of people are missing out on sleep and harming their brains in the process.

The obvious answer is to limit your smartphone use for when you really need it. But there are other things you can do.

Download a free blue-lighter filtering app like Twilight or Blue Light Filter from your phone's app store.

Get a 25% Brain Boost with This *Forbidden* Dessert

It feels like the older we get, everything involving our brains gets a little bit harder.

Things we used to take for granted like remembering names, balancing our check books, or keeping our schedules straight become more and more of a challenge.

So if you heard there was a natural substance that could give you a 25 percent brain boost, you probably couldn't sign up fast enough.

Well, the good news is that this substance exists—but your doctor has probably been telling you for years to stay away from it.

This miracle brain-booster is cocoa—as in real, natural cocoa, not the sugar-loaded processed junk in the supermarket candy aisle. And it's loaded with healthy compounds that could have you thinking and remembering better than ever.

In a landmark study from Columbia University Medical Center, researchers divided healthy adults aged 50 to 69 into two groups.

The first group drank a solution with flavonols extracted

from cocoa. Flavonols are micronutrients found in plant-based foods (quercetin is a well-known example) and they've been proven to promote brain and heart health.

The second group drank little or none.

After just three months, the research team tested both groups on memory tasks and measured blood flow in certain areas of the brain. Those who drank the cocoa flavonols performed about 25 percent better than the control group.

Imagine that—a 25 percent brain boost from a healthy, delicious treat that most seniors are being told is bad for them. Just more bum health advice from the mainstream!

And, believe it or not, the wonders of cocoa don't end there.

Dr. Giulio Maria Pasinetti is a professor of neurology at the Icahn School of Medicine at Mount Sinai, and he's spent his career studying the powers of cocoa and cocoa extracts.

Through animal studies and his research on polyphenols, micronutrients in cocoa that are known to reduce age-related cognitive decline, Dr. Pasinetti has developed a fascinating theory.

He believes that cocoa helps inhibit the development of toxic proteins, such as the beta-amyloid plaque that is found in the brains of people with Alzheimer's disease.

Beta-amyloid proteins cause loss of synapses, the connections between brain cells that allow electrical and chemical signals to pass from one cell to another. Cocoa may also help the brain clear out these proteins once they're generated.

In fact, a study out of Tufts University found that people with diabetes and hypertension, two major risk factors for dementia, improved blood flow to their brains and cognitive function after just one month of drinking two cups of cocoa a day.

Let's see the drug companies produce results like that!

In choosing a cocoa, go for cocoa that has not been 'dutched,' a treatment with alkali used to make cocoa darker and less acidic. Rapunzel Organic Cocoa Powder is a good option. You can pick it up at **www.iherb.com**.

Chinese Breakthrough REVERSES Alzheimer's in 8 Weeks

It's Practically Unknown in America...But It's PROVEN to Improve Brain Function 60%

You've spent your entire life building up precious memories... of weddings, childbirths, anniversaries, and so much more.

But Alzheimer's doesn't care about any of that, does it?

It steals a lifetime of memories, one by one. It steals your personality, and what it means to be you.

And finally it steals your independence...and even your life.

But it doesn't have to be this way. *Not for you or the people you love.*

Because there's an ancient Chinese compound that attacks the actual cause of your Alzheimer's and memory problems.

In fact, it's been proven to **reverse the symptoms of Alzheimer's in just 8 weeks.**

Big Pharma has been trying to copy it for decades, with drugs like Aricept, Exelon, and Razadyne.

But you can get your hands on the real deal...this memory-restoring Chinese moss...*right now.*

Just don't expect to hear about it at ANY mainstream doctor's office.

The Alzheimer's Cure Doctors Have NEVER Heard Of

Huperzine A is a very special compound found in an ancient moss (called *Huperzia serrata*) that grows throughout China.

For centuries, Chinese healers have used this moss to protect their brains and think more clearly.

Now, it looks like Huperzine A is the Alzheimer's breakthrough we've all been waiting for.

You, *huperzine A is a natural nootropic.* That means it works directly on your brain to improve function and memory.

How does it work?

Huperzine A increases levels of the neurotransmitter acetylcholine in your brain by blocking the action of the enzyme cholinesterase.

This can all get a little scientific, but here are the two things you need to know.

#1: Cholinesterase builds up in your brain over time and disrupts the communication between nerve cells. That triggers Alzheimer's and other forms of dementia.

#2: Acetylcholine delivers messages within your brain, and helps you form new memories and think more clearly.

So LESS cholinesterase and MORE acetylcholine means LESS Alzheimer's. Simple as that.

And that's exactly what huperzine A does.

But it doesn't stop here.

Additionally, **huperzine A works to protect your brain's neurons from damage due to toxins like peroxides, beta-amyloids, and glutamate.**

Believe it or not, Big Pharma has been trying to imitate the effects of huperzine A with Alzheimer's drugs for ages.

But these meds come with a big problem.

These so-called cholinesterase inhibitors increase acetylcholine all over your body, which can cause issues with the GI tract, lungs, muscles, and more.

Huperzine A, on the other hand, doesn't have these problems because it only affects the cholinesterase and acetylcholine in your brain.

So it's safer and more effective – and doesn't come with all the side effects.

In fact, it's now been **scientifically proven** to dramatically improve your brain function in just 8 weeks.

Stacking the Benefits of Huperzine A

While huperzine A will deliver incredible brain-boosting benefits on its own, it can yield even greater results by increased *stacking* it with the right additional components.

Stacking refers to the practice of taking multiple supplements that complement one another – either by working together to amp up the benefits or by expediting those benefits within your body.

For instance, taking huperzine A in combination with a choline source like **Alpha GPC** can increase the amount of acetylcholine in the brain, further enhancing the effect of huperzine A.

Another good choice for stacking with huperzine A is a racetam, such as **Pramiracetam**.

Racetams activate receptors that are located near your acetylcholine receptors. This sensitizes your acetylcholine receptors, increasing the potential benefits of huperzine A.

Further, huperzine A can be paired with **Noopept**, a powerful and popular nootropic.

Nootropics, like racetams, benefit your cognitive abilities and act to protect your brain.

But, unlike other nootropics that can take days, weeks, or

even months to kick in, the effects of Noopept can be felt almost immediately after ingestion.

So, if you're interested in getting even more out of taking huperzine A, consider *stacking* your supplements!

58% Improvement in Just 8 Weeks

The evidence supporting huperzine A for Alzheimer's is overwhelming.

In fact, a review of 20 randomized controlled trials shows that **huperzine A has an incredibly positive effect on brain function and quality of life for people with Alzheimer's disease.**

In 1995, when huperzine A was still a relatively new concept to Western researchers, a double-blind study from Zhejiang Medical University in China quickly revealed its impressive capabilities.

The study involved 103 Alzheimer's patients – 50 received 200mcg of huperzine A and the other 53 received a placebo, every day for 8 weeks.

Throughout the research, the participants were given regular memory exams, including the Wechsler memory scale and the mini-mental state examination (MMSE) scale.

If you or someone you love has Alzheimer's, you may be familiar with both of these tests.

At the end of the 8 weeks, **58 percent of the patients** treated with huperzine A showed **significant improvements** in memory, thinking, and behavioral functions.

That's literally life-changing.

In a more recent study, huperzine A was tested on 202 Alzheimer's patients at the Peking Medical College Hospital in China.

One group was given 400mcg of huperzine A each day for 12 weeks while the other group was given a placebo.

At the end of the study, the group treated v
A showed remarkable improvement in cogni
and mood, in comparison to the placebo grou

And these are just two of many incredible st

What's more? Huperzine A has also been studied as a memory enhancer for people with healthy brains.

So, you don't have to be suffering from Alzheimer's or dementia to enjoy the benefits of this remarkable supplement. You simply have to want a brain boost.

Even more impressive? Some people can feel a change after a single dose of Huperzine A!

The Natural Way to Beat Alzheimer's

Huperzine A is used all over China – but it's practically unknown in America.

And drug companies want to keep it that way.

Fortunately, huperzine A supplements are available at many health food stores and can be easily found online.

Some of the best options are tablets from manufacturers like **Life Extention** and supplements from specialized nootropic vendors like **AbsorbYourHealth.com**.

Experts recommend taking up to 200mcg twice a day to treat Alzheimer's and at least 50mcg for Alzheimer's and dementia prevention.

Additionally, it is advised that you take huperzine A daily for three weeks and then take 5-7 days off to avoid developing a dependency.

With the right dosage and regimen, huperzine A can bring you or your loved one back from the edge of dementia – and that's *nothing short of a miracle.*

African Seed Fights Depression Better Than Prozac

Underground Treatment Begins Relieving Symptoms in 2 Hours?!

Suffering from depression can feel like spending every day in a nightmare.

You can't relax…you lose interest in relationships and activities you used to love…and maybe some days you don't even feel like getting out of bed.

And your blues are big business for the drug companies.

They're making a fortune selling selective-serotonin reuptake inhibitors (SSRIs) like Paxil and Prozac that can make you gain weight, weaken your bones, and *even destroy your sex life!*

And mainstream doctors will tell you it's the only way to finally get control of your depression.

But that's simply not true.

Because there's a powerful African seed that's **now running circles around prescription drugs** for beating depression and anxiety.

It's safe…backed by years of science…and it's been proven to start delivering relief in as little as two hours.

The Serotonin Secret

If you suffer from depression or anxiety, you've probably heard a thing or two about serotonin.

It's a key neurotransmitter that's vital to your brain…and when you don't make enough of it, problems like depression, anxiety, and even insomnia set in.

Lots of the SSRI medications on the market target serotonin—**but these drugs come with the BIG problem.**

All they do is help the little serotonin in your brain stick around and work a bit longer.

That's like wringing a dry sponge!

If you want to beat depression and other mood disorders, you need to help your body make MORE serotonin.

That's just common sense, right?

"5-HTP is a safe and effective alternative to prescription antidepressants."

And that's where a plant called *Griffonia simplicifolia* comes into the picture.

Griffonia simplicifolia is a small, climbing plant that grows throughout Africa and bears greenish flowers that then transform into black pods full of seeds.

Natives have use the seeds for centuries to treat everything from sexual dysfunction (which is also linked to low serotonin) to digestive problems.

But now it looks like *Griffonia simplicifolia* is the natural depression breakthrough we've all been waiting for.

That's because it's loaded with 5-hydroxytryptophan—aka 5-HTP—a critical amino acid that's related to tryptophan, an amino acid found in high-protein foods like poultry, seafood, dairy, and eggs.

More importantly, **your body needs 5-HTP to make serotonin!**

5-HTP easily crosses your blood-brain barrier, where it can help make the serotonin your brain needs to fight depression and anxiety.

The formula is simple—**more 5-HTP means MORE serotonin**. And that means less depression for you.

And research is now proving that if you suffer from depression, loading up on 5-HTP should be the FIRST thing you try.

Running Circles Around Prozac

Doctors write so many prescriptions for Prozac that it's a wonder they don't develop carpal tunnel syndrome.

But they should be recommending 5-HTP instead.

In a landmark study on patients with clinical depression and anxiety, *5-HTP reduced symptoms just as well as Prozac*, but with far fewer side effects.

For my money, **that makes 5-HTP BETTER than Prozac... and safer.**

Another study compared the effects of 5-HTP to the antidepressant Luvox.

It found that, of the 63 participants, those who were given 5-HTP did just as well as those who received Luvox for a mood disorder.

Again, with fewer side effects.

Even better, 5-HTP goes to work lightning-fast—unlike prescription antidepressants that can take weeks to kick in.

In one study, 48 patients with panic disorders were given either a 200 mg capsule of 5-HTP or a placebo.

Just 90 minutes later, all participants were subjected to a CO_2 "challenge" in which they inhaled air rich in carbon dioxide to induce panic attacks.

The folks who took 5-HTP were much less likely to suffer from anxiety and panic attacks.

Anxiety relief in less than two hours!

And that just makes sense, because research has shown that your intestines can absorb more than 50 percent of the 5-HTP you ingest in about 90 minutes.

In other words, it does to work FAST.

Where to Get 5-HTP

If you suffer from depression, anxiety or both, there's a good chance you have naturally low levels of 5-HTP.

Correcting this deficiency with a supplement could be the key to unlocking depression relief that you didn't even know was possible!

Research recommends 200 mg daily as a safe and beneficial dose to best increase serotonin in the brain.

You can find 100 mg tablets from **Nature's Bounty** as well as **Thorne Research**.

In just 90 minutes, this miraculous compound made from rare African seeds will have already increased your serotonin levels.

All for a fraction of the cost of SSRIs and with none of the side effects.

You have nothing to lose…and a whole lot to gain.

4 More Benefits of 5-HTP

1. Eases chronic pain

In a double-blind, placebo-controlled study, researchers gave 100 mg of 5-HTP to 50 fibromyalgia patients over a 30-day period. At the end of the study, the patients reported a significant decrease in tenderness, pain, insomnia, and anxiety. There are still many unanswered questions about fibromyalgia, but it's been shown that patients have lower levels of serotonin.

2. Helps with diet and weight loss

Carbohydrates increase serotonin levels in the brain and create a sense of addiction. Instead, 5-HTP can mitigates those craving by increasing serotonin without eating carbs. In clinical trials, 5-HTP supplementation in obese women resulted in no mood changes but decreased food intake and weight loss

3. 5-HTP helps alleviate Type II Diabetes

In a clinical trial involving 25 overweight diabetics, subjects who received 5-HTP had reduced caloric, carbohydrate, and fat intake compared to a placebo. Subjects who received 5-HTP also had reduced body weight, blood sugar, insulin, and HbA1C levels after two week.

4. 5-HTP improves sleep quality

Genetic mutations can cause serotonin deficiencies which cause people to overeat. This increased appetite upsets the circadian rhythm that allows for sound sleep. But, with 5-HTP supplementation, normal circadian rhythm and food intake can be restored. One clinical trial demonstrated that the use of 5-HTP significantly improved sleep quality in 9 subjects with sleep disorders.

IGNORED Asian Cure Boosts Brain Power in 2 Hours Flat

It Lifts Brain Fog, Erases Stress, and Helps You Think More Clearly

Earlier in this issue, I talked about the powerful MEND Program—and how it's delivering amazing results for people with Alzheimer's disease.

But let's face it…not all the problems with our brains are as serious as Alzheimer's.

Maybe you're just having more of those "senior moments," where you keep losing your wallet or can't remember where you parked your car.

Or maybe you just want to be able to focus and think more clearly, like you did 10 or even 20 years ago.

Well, believe it or not, the Chinese have been sitting on one of the most powerful brain boosters around for 2,000 years.

But odds are, you've never heard about it.

Because this is one health breakthrough that even natural doctors are ignoring.

The Ancient Secret to a Quiz-Show Brain

It seems like adaptogens are all the rage these days—and with good reason.

These natural remedies help wipe away stress and reset your hormone levels. And that can have MAJOR benefits for your brain.

But the natural medicine community has become completely obsessed with hot-selling adaptogens like ashwagandha and rhodiola.

And it seems like they've forgotten all about the powers of the simple schisandra berry.

In fact, schisandra (known as Wu Wei Zu in China) is practically unknown outside of its home country!

And that's a big mistake, when you consider all the brain-healthy nutrients packed into every berry, including:

- Powerful antioxidants like dihydropaseic acid and isoscoparin;
- Melatonin, a sleep aid tied to better brain performance;
- Quercetin, an anti-inflammatory and proven brain-booster;
- Essential nutrients like vitamins C and E, as well as nickel, copper, magnesium, and zinc;
- And much, much more!

"Schisandra enjoys millennia of traditional use for slowing the aging process, increasing energy, as a fatigue-fighter, and as a sexual tonic."

The Chinese regularly use schisandra in stews, and it's considered so important that there's even a research institute dedicated to it in the Lioaning Province!

And once you understand what schisandra can do for your

brain, you're going to be researching (and buying) it yourself.

In fact, it's now been proven to help you ***think better and more clearly in just two hours flat!***

Two Hours to a Better, Faster, Stronger Brain

Schisandra goes to work increasing your brain function in three powerful ways:

Brain Booster #1: Even a small dose of schisandra reduces your levels of cortisol, a key stress hormone linked to cognitive performance. This allows your body to calm down, think clearly, and cope with mental and physical stress.

Brain Booster #2: Schisandra optimizes your brain's levels of both norepinephrine (a nervous system hormone) and dopamine (a vital neurotransmitter). That increases the ability to maintain focus and improves mood.

Brain Booster #3: Schisandra normalizes metabolic pathways throughout the entire body, which helps fight against stress, anxiety, depression, and fatigue.

Schisandra is backed by thousands of years of use—but when American researchers put it to the test, they were blown away by the results.

It started boosting brain function in just two hours!

A team from the National Institutes of Health analyzed mental performance for a group of women—half were given schisandra and half weren't.

The participants were given something called the Stroop Colour-Word test before and after taking schisandra.

Basically, this test measures your ability to think clearly and accurately—even when you're faced with stress, interference, interruptions, etc.

And after just two hours, the women who received schisandra were performing off the charts!

They were paying attention better...answering questions

faster…and they were making fewer mistakes.

It was is *someone had given their brains a tune-up!*

Imagine what that kind of difference could mean in YOUR life.

How to Get Your Hands on Schisandra

Many doctors (including natural ones) may have forgotten about schisandra—but getting your hands on it is still easy enough.

If you have access to a Chinese grocery store or medicine shop, you may be able to find dried schisandra berries.

Just a few berries added to your diet every day is enough to reap all the benefits.

Berries can also be purchased online through **Bulk Apothecary** and **Live Superfoods**.

Better still, you can easily buy schisandra as a supplement online through suppliers like **Swanson Health**.

It comes in 500 mg. doses and will cost you less than $10 a month.

Schisandra Benefits
1. Lowers Inflammation

Thanks to it's high concentration of antioxidant compounds, schisandra helps fight free radical damage and lowers inflammatory responses.

2. Supports Adrenal Function and Lowers Stress

Known as an adaptogenic agent, schisandra helps balance hormones and therefore improves our ability to deal with stressors, both physical and psychological.

3. Improves Liver Function and Digestive Health

Schisandra helps increase enzyme production, boosts antioxidant activity, and improves circulation, digestion and the ability to remove waste from the body.

4. Protects the Skin

Schisandra is a natural beauty tonic that's capable of protecting the skin from wind, sun exposure, allergic reactions, dermatitis, environmental stress and toxin accumulation.

5. Improves Mental Performance

Studies also show a link between schisandra use and protection against neurological and psychiatric disorders.

6. Helps with Healthy Sexual Function

Research shows that schisandra is beneficial for fertility and hormonal health because it positively impacts hormone production.

MEND Program Turns Back Alzheimer's in 3 Months?!?

It's the Holy Grail of the pharmaceutical industry…a magic pill that can reverse Alzheimer's, one of the most tragic diseases of aging.

For years the largest drug companies on Earth have tried to develop an Alzheimer's medication that works—and for years they've failed.

And science is now proving that there may be a very good reason for that. Because while many drugs try to attack Alzheimer's in just one way, it turns out that the disease isn't so simple.

The fact is, there are many contributing factors that can lead to an Alzheimer's diagnosis—such as inflammation, dysfunction in our mitochondria (the energy centers for our cells, including brain cells), abnormal hormone levels, and much more.

If you want to beat Alzheimer's, you need an approach that tackles all of these causes at their source. And some brilliant scientists at UCLA may have just found it.

In fact, they have now developed…

A powerful Alzheimer's CURE that goes to work in just 3 months!

Imagine a lifetime of memories...your personality...even your ability to live independently starting to return in as little as 90 days! Picture that brain fog lifting, and being able to think clearly for the first time in ages.

It's not just possible...it's actually happening for people just like you, whose situations seemed completely hopeless.

These results are being delivered by something called the MEND Program, which stands for metabolic enhancement for neurodegeneration.

The program focuses on restoring metabolic and hormonal imbalances, and giving your brain the fuel it needs to operate like it did years ago.

The protocol was published by UCLA researchers in 2014, and the results are turning conventional thinking about Alzheimer's on its head.

And it should, when you consider people like Mary, who had their lives changed by the MEND Program.

Mary was 67 years old and had been suffering serious memory problems for two years. She couldn't perform her job and was going to have to quit—and she was even having trouble driving and navigating roads.

But after just three months on the MEND Program, her symptoms were gone!

That's right—memory loss completely reversed in just 90 days!

And Mary isn't alone. Of the 10 people studied in the UCLA research—all with varying levels of memory loss—nine experienced substantial improvements. **A 90% success rate!**

The MEND Program is something you need to do under the guidance of a physician—and each program is personalized based on your lab work and other health conditions.

But there are some key elements of the program that are fairly consistent, such as:

- A prescribed diet, such as a low-glycemic or anti-inflammation eating plan. High blood sugar and inflammation are both heavily linked to several degenerative diseases, such as Alzheimer's. So you follow a diet designed to attack these problems.

- Optimizing sleep, using natural supplements like melatonin, as needed. The goal is to get a solid 8 hours of sleep every night. A lack of sleep is a significant contributor to cognitive decline.

- An exercise program of 30-60 minutes a day, 4-6 times a week. Regular exercise has also been proven to help reduce the risk of memory loss.

- Supplements like B12 to reduce levels of homocysteine, a major contributor to Alzheimer's.

- Prebiotics or probiotics to clear up digestive issues, which can trigger inflammation and other autoimmune problems.

- Brain fuel, such as coconut oil. Coconut oil contains medium-chain triglycerides, which your brain can use as an alternative source of fuel if your brain cells have trouble with glucose.

- Regulating hormone levels, such as cortisol, which can contribute to cognitive decline.

MEND takes a disciplined and multi-faceted approach to treating Alzheimer's. But because so many factors contribute to this disease, this is exactly what you need.

And while it takes some work to stick to a MEND Program, with a 90% success rate, it's a protocol that's well worth following.

The biggest drawback to MEND is that it's new and many doctors may not know about it. And let's face it—lots of mainstream docs have been practically trained to give up on Alzheimer's patients.

But this is something you can take into your own hands. Muses Labs, out of Raleigh, NC, actually works with physicians and helps them implement the MEND Program for patients like you.

You can learn more about Muses Labs at **www.museslabs.com**. There's even a place on the website where your doctor can contact a Muses Labs professional directly for more information about the program.

Can This "Virgin Mary Secret" Restore Lost Memory?

It's been said that all the wisdom of the world can be found in the pages of the Holy Bible.

And it seems like year after year, scientists are proving this is true.

We're learning that our Creator has filled Earth with miraculous, natural treatments for the worst diseases of aging, like dementia, heart disease, arthritis, diabetes, and even cancer.

Many of these breakthroughs can be found right in the pages of the Bible…or have connections to the most important figures in Christianity.

Earlier in this report, you learned about the MEND Program, developed at UCLA, that takes a multi-faceted approach to treating dementia and Alzheimer's at the source.

Now, researchers believe they've also discovered a revolutionary, Biblically-based herb that can attack one of the greatest contributors to dementia and Alzheimer's…and **maybe even reverse years of memory loss!**

It's called milk thistle…or the "Virgin Mary Flower"…and the research behind it is leaving brain scientists and Christians absolutely speechless!

The story behind milk thistle is the stuff of legend. The plant produces a beautiful purple flower with pure white veins.

For years it's been claimed that milk thistle got its white accents when a drop of milk from the Virgin Mary fell on the plant while she was nursing the infant Jesus. And now research has proven that...

Milk thistle is a medical miracle, delivered straight from our Creator Himself!

The story starts when British researchers focused on a specific family of proteins found within your cells called carbonic anhydrase I and II.

It turns out that these proteins are in far greater quantity in older brains, and in young brains that had become sick with early onset decay and degeneration.

The more protein was present, the older the brain behaved.

What's worse, when they injected the protein into young, healthy brains...it turned them old.

But here's the thing—if you can target this protein, stop it from forming, and flush it from your system, you may be able to **stop degenerative diseases like Alzheimer's and dementia right in their tracks.**

And here's the good news—the miraculous compound that blocks the very specific forms of carbonic anhydrase is the ALL-NATURAL extract from milk thistle.

The British research team even concluded that milk thistle extract "is a good inhibitor of carbonic anhydrase forms called CA I and CA II."

And these scientists aren't the only ones jumping on the bandwagon as far as milk thistle...the powerful Virgin Mary Flower...is concerned. The world-renowned Mayo Clinic wrote that milk thistle extract "demonstrated a beneficial effect on people with various neurodegenerative disorders, including multiple sclerosis (MS), Parkinson's disease, and Alzheimer's disease."

Plus, there's this from the Susan G. Komen Foundation:

"Early research suggests that taking a combination supplement containing [milk thistle extract] improves mental function in people with Alzheimer's disease."

Improving mental function in people with Alzheimer's disease! How many drugs on the market today can claim THAT?!?

Imagine watching brain fog lift and memories return, thanks to this powerful natural remedy! Instead of fighting against these natural treatments…given to us by our loving Creator… our government should be shouting about them from the rooftops!

But we know that with the Feds in Big Pharma's pocket, that's never going to happen. And that's a shame for millions of Americans, because hundreds of studies are turning up more powerful uses for milk thistle.

Here's what the National Cancer Institute has published on what milk thistle is capable of doing…

- Has direct anti-cancer effects against prostate, breast, colon, skin and cervical cancer…
- Boosts the regrowth of liver tissue…
- Destroys free radicals…
- Stops bone loss…
- Decreases cholesterol…
- Reduces inflammation…

You don't need to wait for Uncle Sam to come to his senses to put milk thistle to work for you.

You can buy Puritan's Pride 1,000 mg milk thistle extract for around $10 a month at **www.puritan.com**.

CHAPTER 9:

BANISH COLDS, FEVERS AND FLU WITH THESE FORGOTTEN MEDICAL MARVELS

7 Hay Fever Breakthroughs Big Pharma Doesn't Want You to Know About

They say April showers bring May flowers.

But if you suffer from hay fever, that's not all the spring and summer months bring. They bring congestion, running noses, sneezing, coughing, and lots of other miserable allergy symptoms.

And that's when the drug companies start running their round-the-clock commercials for heavy-duty drugs that come with a long list of side effects.

Especially if you take corticosteroid nasal sprays, you could be dealing with headaches, bloody noses, and even potentially serious infections.

Who needs all that? Especially when there are underground natural remedies that can help relieve some of the worst hay fever symptoms.

Hay Fever Fighter #1: Honey

It is believed that honey helps hay fever because you become desensitized by the bee pollen in the honey. If you gradually increase the amount of honey that you eat, you will probably be able to feel much better pretty quickly. When using the honey, make sure you use some that is local because that is what will desensitize you to the local pollen around you.

Hay Fever Fighter #2: Vitamin C

Vitamin C is a well-known, natural antihistamine and is found in lemons, grapefruit and oranges. It also contains bioflavonoids, which can have a strong anti-allergenic effect. By combining vitamin C and bioflavonoids, you will have a terrific natural decongestant and antihistamine to help you get rid of your symptoms.

If you don't want to eat the fruit, you can always take vitamin C supplements, which are available everywhere. Usually about 1,000 mg. per day is an effective dose.

Hay Fever Fighter #3: Hot peppers

There is an active element called capsaicin in both red and chili peppers. When these are eaten, the nasal passages are opened up and the congestion that usually goes along with hay fever is reduced.

Capsaicin is also available as a supplement. Go to **www.iherb.com** for plenty of capsaicin supplement options.

Hay Fever Fighter #4: Carotenoids

These are pigments that are found in plants naturally. They act as strong antioxidants, reducing the inflammation in airways and improving the immune system.

You will find carotenoids in foods that are easy to add to your diet, like apricots, carrots, spinach, pumpkin and sweet potatoes.

Hay Fever Fighter #5: Chamomile tea

Chamomile tea is both an antihistamine and an antioxidant. It contains flavonoids and it can be an effective anti-inflammatory agent. You can either drink this tea or you can use it as a compress on your eyes. It will have a soothing, cooling effect and will help your red, swollen and irritable eyes feel better.

Hay Fever Fighter #6: Garlic

Believe it or not, using garlic in your diet can help improve your immune system. It is also a great decongestant and helps to ease many of the minor symptoms of hay fever.

Garlic acts as an anti-inflammatory and is a great source of quercetin, which is a natural antihistamine. You can either eat raw or crushed garlic. If that doesn't sound appealing, you can take a garlic capsule (**www.iherb.com** is a great source for buying supplements).

Hay fever fighter #7: Onions

Onion skins contain a great deal of quercetin, the anti-inflammatory and antihistamine mentioned above.

Onions are particularly useful because they have three times the amount of quercetin as kale and 10 times more than broccoli. Best of all, they can be eaten at any time of day, in a variety of meals.

All of these remedies are perfectly safe, and they can make a big difference in your fight against hay fever.

How to Make Your Own Cough Syrup—for *Just a Couple Bucks!*

Buying cold medicine is a little like playing Russian roulette—you never know what you're going to get, or how dangerous it could be.

And some of the cough syrups sold at your local pharmacy are especially risky for people with heart conditions. The good news is that there's a simple cough syrup you can make on your own—and it contains a powerful berry that's been used in folk medicine for centuries.

It's the elderberry, and it's been used in traditional healing in North America, Europe, Asia and Africa.

In particular, the bioflavonoids contained in elderberries are useful in combating viruses that cause colds and flu. In fact, elderberries were used to treat people who became ill during the Panama flu epidemic of 1995.

More recently, elderberry can be found listed in the Mosby's Nursing Drug Reference as a treatment for colds, flu, asthma, congestion, hay fever, and yeast infections. Of course, you'll probably never hear about that from a typical mainstream doctor.

It's easy to make your own elderberry cough syrup at home,

and you may already have a lot of the ingredients.

You can have a good-tasting and effective cold remedy for just a couple dollars a batch. Here's how:

Ingredients:

- 1 cup fresh organic elderberries (1/2 cup dried can be substituted)
- 3 cups purified water
- ¾ cup organic honey
- 1 cinnamon stick
- ½ tsp. ginger
- 2 whole cloves

Step 1: In a saucepan, bring berries, spices, and water to a boil. Reduce heat and simmer for 30 minutes until thick.

Step 2: Smash the berries and strain the mixtures. Let cool.

Step 3: Add honey and stir well.

Store this cough syrup in the refrigerator and it can last for up to three months.

This syrup is safe for children over 12 months. Any product made with honey is not safe for children under a year.

Lower Stubborn Fevers with These Folk Healers' Secrets

When a fever strikes, the first thing lots of people do is to start popping aspirin.

But with all the serious effects that aspirin can have on your gastrointestinal tract, this isn't the best alternative for many people—including seniors.

Fortunately, alternative doctors regularly use a variety of herbs and natural oils to help break fevers. And these treatments are easy to use yourself at home (and if you need to buy them, go to **www.iherb.com**).

Peppermint is a powerful fever-reducing herb. Peppermint essential oil can be used for fast fever reduction by applying it on the forehead, the bottoms of the feet, and along the spine.

It is best to dilute an essential oil in a carrier oil (coconut oil, olive oil, etc.) before applying it directly to the skin. Peppermint tea with lemon and raw local honey is another easy way to get this remedy into your system.

Peppermint can interfere with iron absorption, so use sparingly if the ill person is anemic.

Another option is to take a bath in Epsom salt and chamomile. This is more of a relaxant, but feeling relaxed can go a long way in helping the body to heal.

Chamomile is related to ragweed. It is best to avoid this herb if the ill person has a ragweed allergy.

Rosemary is another herb that can be used for fever reduction. It can be used as an essential oil, infused herbal oil, and a tea, much like with peppermint.

Echinacea is a powerful herbal antibiotic that can be purchased as a supplement. It is often used as a tincture when treating a fever.

Tinctures can be purchased from an herbalist, herbal apothecaries, and health food stores. Nature's Way makes an echinacea tincture that's widely available for less than $10 (just Google Nature's Way echinacea).

Finally, the spice thyme is an excellent herb to use in treating a fever. It can be taken in tincture form, essential oil, and infused herbal oil form.

It can also be blended with Epsom salt and rosemary to make a relaxing and healing herb bath.

Never Get the Flu (or a Flu Shot) Again

It happens like clockwork every year. Once fall hits, we're bombarded with TV commercials and ads at our local doctors' offices and pharmacies telling us to get a flu shot.

The mainstream will even tell you that the flu shot is the only way to make sure you don't come down with a serious case of flu.

Well, you'd normally have to go to a farm to see hogwash like that. The fact is, flu shots are billion-dollar business and our government spends a fortune stockpiling vaccines.

That means they have a vested financial interest in getting you to roll up your sleeve for a shot.

And, believe it or not, that's not even the worst secret as far as the flu shot is concerned. Even if you manage to avoid the side effects (like headache, nausea, and even shoulder injuries from poorly administered vaccines), the flu shot is like playing craps.

It's based on nothing more than a guess on which flu strains will be circulating during a given year—and lots of times, the drug companies guess wrong.

In fact, some years the flu vaccine has been more than 90 percent ineffective for seniors! Who wants odds like that?

Luckily, there are some safe, natural ways to boost your immune system and keep flu from striking. That means no more gambling with that risky flu shot year after year.

The first natural flu-fighter is vitamin D, the so-called "sunshine vitamin." And a study on children (who pass around flu like crazy) found that those who took 1,200 IUs a day were less likely to come down with flu than those who didn't.

Many of us are deficient in vitamin D, especially during the winter months when our bodies have less sunlight to make it naturally. But vitamin D supplements are affordable and easy to pick up at your local drugstore or just about any big-box retailer.

The second natural flu fighter is the mineral zinc. Our bodies need zinc for our immune systems to work properly, and loading up on zinc just makes sense during cold and flu season.

After all, studies have shown that people with weaker immune systems are more likely to develop flu—or to get more serious cases of it.

An Italian study on seniors showed that zinc can naturally boost your body's natural supply of white blood cells that you need to fight off infections, like flu.

Zinc supplements are widely available, but you can also load up on foods that are rich in zinc. Some of the best are spinach, beef, shrimp, and even pumpkin seeds.

Finally, the mineral selenium is shaping up to be an important flu fighter. In fact, an animal study out of the University of North Carolina, Chapel Hill found that being deficient in selenium (as many people are) can force flu viruses to mutate into more serious forms.

"We believe our latest findings are both important and potentially disturbing because they suggest nutritional deficiencies can promote epidemics in a way not appreciated before," Dr. Melinda A. Beck, the lead author, said.

Foods like Brazil nuts, yellowfin tuna, sardines, and even chicken are excellent sources of selenium.

There are also supplements that combine several of these flu fighters. Carlson Lab's ACES + Zn has both zinc and selenium, and you can pick it up at **www.pureformulas.com.**

Soothe Your Grandkids' Colds _Without_ Dangerous Meds

There's no greater joy than when your children drop off the grandkids for a visit.

But when those grandchildren…especially when they're babies…are sick, that joy can turn into a challenge really fast. It can be a helpless feeling to see our little loved ones suffer from colds, and most store-bought cold remedies are unsafe for infants.

Fortunately, there are plenty of natural treatments for baby colds. Here are some you can try to be a hero to your littlest grandkids (and to their moms and dads).

#1 Stuffy noses

To help your little one clear his nose, provide plenty of liquids. For a small baby, breastmilk or formula is ideal.

Saline drops are very helpful in clearing blocked passages. Getting them into tiny nostrils, however, is easier said than done.

Try using a dropper and have someone else hold the baby

while you put the liquid into the infant's nose. Another option is to swaddle the baby so his hands are restrained.

If some bottled breastmilk has been left for you, it can be a useful alternative. Use a dropper to place one or two drops in each nostril.

Using a special tool like the NoseFrida (you can get it at CVS, WalMart or Target) to suction mucus is particularly helpful for smaller babies. Since infants can't blow their noses or even sniff to clear their nostrils, suction gets some of the mucus out and lets them breathe easier. You can loosen the mucus first with saline drops.

Sleeping upright is also good for stuffy little noses. If you have a firm wedge that can go in the baby's crib, it will hold the baby in the right position to help clear those nasal passages.

#2 Coughs

The type of cough will indicate the treatment. A barking cough can be attributed to croup and the best thing for this is cold air. Take your well bundled baby outdoors for a few minutes in winter to treat. He will breathe in the cold air and this will ease the cough.

In warmer climates or during the summer, opening the freezer and standing in front of it provides similar relief.

For regular coughing fits, steam can be quite beneficial. You may want to try the old method of running a hot shower to fill the bathroom with steam.

You also can try adding a few drops of essential oil to a room diffuser. Lemon, ginger and eucalyptus are all excellent choices for a baby's cold. Never apply these directly to your child's skin.

#3 Fevers

Treating a fever naturally can be frightening. Keep in mind that the fever itself is not bad. It is actually a sign that the baby's body is working to fight off the virus.

That being said, always see a doctor if a baby's temperature is over 104 degrees and the infant is more than three months old. For babies under three months, any fever over 100.4 degrees can be dangerous.

Your little one will need to stay hydrated, so make sure he has plenty of liquids. Breastmilk is good, since it also contains antibodies, but the important thing is to keep liquid intake up.

A cool washcloth, just barely dampened, can also be placed on the back of the neck or on your baby's forehead to bring down a fever. Another option is to wipe his body down with a mixture of water with a little vinegar mixed in.

Finally, lavender essential oil can also be mixed into a carrier oil, such as coconut oil, and gently rubbed on the back of the baby's neck. In many cases, this will help a fever drop or even break completely.

Having a sick infant is never fun, but having a plan in mind can help. Your baby will be more comfortable and you can rest easier, knowing that everything used is natural.

Ancient "Quack" Treatment Provides Allergy Relief

If you suffer from allergies, you've probably tried just about everything looking for relief.

And you've learned the hard way that lots of the prescription and over-the-counter drugs on the market either don't work, or leave you feeling like you have 24-hour brain fog.

It's amazing that many mainstream doctors still don't recommend acupuncture for allergies, even though there's solid evidence behind it. Some even call it a "quack" treatment.

But if you're tired of dealing with daily allergy misery, acupuncture may just be the safe, effective treatment you've been looking for.

Acupuncture is an ancient Chinese medical practice that promotes healing using tiny needles inserted into the skin. It dates back thousands of years.

The needles stimulate nerves which lead back to the brain and spinal cord. According to the University of Maryland Medical Center, acupuncture also increases circulation.

Two major studies have examined acupuncture's role in treating allergies, and the results were outstanding.

The first study tracked 422 allergy sufferers over a period of two months. One group received no acupuncture treatment, a second group received fake acupuncture at non-important points of the body and a third group received real acupuncture according to traditional Chinese practices.

Study leaders told participants to take oral antihistamines as needed to control their allergy symptoms. At the end of the study, participants reported on their use of oral medication. The participants who received real acupuncture took the least amount of medication for their allergy symptoms.

Imagine better allergy control, without having to rely on those potentially dangerous medications. Sounds good, right?

Another smaller study, published in the *American Journal of Chinese Medicine*, reported that acupuncture reduced allergy symptoms in all participants.

That's right—*a 100 percent success rate.*

Even better, the study noted that participants did not report any adverse side effects from the treatment.

Many alternative doctors are using acupuncture right now to help patients control their allergies. But when it comes to seeking treatment, not all acupuncturists are created equally.

You want to get an acupuncturist with the highest level of training. Your best bet is to visit the website for the American Academy of Medical Acupuncture at **www.medicalacupuncture. org.**

The website has a search function that will help you find licensed medical acupuncturists near you.

5 More Cold Remedies Sitting in Your Pantry Right Now

Nothing is more miserable than a cough that will not quit. When you are suffering from one, the last thing you want to do is drive out to the drugstore to pick up cough medicine.

Worse still, many commercial cough remedies are expensive, can cause uncomfortable side effects, or contain substances, like alcohol, that are not recommended for some patients.

Never fear. You probably have everything you need to soothe your cough right in your kitchen cabinets. Here are five natural substances that can provide you with instant, safe, and inexpensive relief:

Cold Remedy #1: Honey

As we discussed earlier, honey is also great for controlling stubborn allergies.

Studies have shown honey to be as effective in relieving a cough as over-the-counter medicines. Honey is a natural antiseptic as well as a soothing agent. Take a couple of teaspoons in your tea, or mix it in hot water with some of the other ingredients discussed below.

Take honey as often as you need it. There are no ill effects from too much of nature's best sweetener.

Cold Remedy #2: Ginger

Some natural health practitioners refer to ginger as the "universal medicine" because it has been shown to calm the digestive system, stimulate the circulatory system, and prevent respiratory tract ailments.

For a cough, sip commercially available ginger tea or grate about an inch of a fresh ginger root into a teapot of boiling water. Adding a little honey and lemon will enhance the soothing effect.

Cold Remedy #3: Lemon

Lemons are rich in vitamin C and other vitamins and minerals as well as having antiseptic, astringent, and antioxidant properties.

An old remedy for a cough is to suck on a salted slice of lemon. If the thought of that sends you into a perpetual pucker, then just squeeze some lemon juice into a mug of boiling water or warm up a glass of lemonade.

Cold Remedy #4: Apple cider vinegar

Apple cider vinegar is a powerful antimicrobial, which, when ingested, creates an alkaline environment in the body that helps kills bacteria and viruses.

A tablespoon of apple cider vinegar a day, straight up or mixed in a glass of water, may help benefit colds, weight management, and even blood sugar. When combined with some of the other ingredients on this list, apple cider vinegar is an effective cough suppression tonic.

Cold Remedy #5: Cayenne pepper

For the brave, a tonic made from the recipe below uses the expectorant properties of cayenne peppers to suppress and sooth coughs. Mix it up in a jar and take a spoonful as often as you need to.

- 1 tsp ground cayenne pepper
- 1 tsp ground ginger
- ¼ cup cider vinegar
- ½ cup water
- ¼ cup honey

You should always check with your doctor about a cough that lasts more than two weeks. But if you are simply seeking relief from the cough of a common cold, why not turn first to your pantry, and try one of these natural and safe alternatives to commercial cough medicines?

Stop Sore Throat Pain in Just Seconds with These Proven Helpers

When you have a sore throat, you just want it gone fast. But lots of the drug store remedies either don't provide enough relief, or can only be used every couple hours or so.

Who wants to sit around waiting to feel better?

Fortunately, there are plenty of "kitchen cures" that can soothe a sore throat—and you'll feel them working in just seconds.

Sore Throat Soother #1: Honey

There's a reason you keep seeing honey as a remedy for cold and allergy symptoms—it works!

Honey contains a lot of vitamins and helps boost your immune system. Add a teaspoon of honey to some hot water and drink it at night, or add it to tea during the day, instead of sugar.

It might also be helpful to add lemon juice to the nighttime water mix. Lemon juice has an astringent effect, which helps in both shrinking the mucous membranes and in getting rid of bacteria and viruses that may be responsible for your sore throat.

Sore Throat Soother #2: Turmeric

The spice turmeric (and its active ingredient curcumin) is renowned for being a powerful antioxidant and can have beneficial effects for a sore throat.

Mix a half-teaspoon of turmeric with one teaspoon of salt in a cup of hot water. Don't swallow! Gargle this solution to get rid of the bacteria and reduce irritation in your throat.

Sore Throat Soother #3: Cloves

Cloves are a potent antibacterial spice that not only smell and taste wonderful, but can be useful when it comes to relieving a sore throat. Use two teaspoons of powdered cloves mixed into warm water.

Gargle the solution to calm the irritation in your throat and also reduce the amount of bacteria in your mouth.

Oil of cloves can be used in place of the powdered version, or you can even chew the spice in its natural form for both antibacterial and anesthetic effects.

Sore Throat Soother #4: Licorice root

Licorice root is a powerful antibacterial that can be useful for sore throat relief. You can mix it with water and gargle as often as needed. The root is sold in both powdered and extract forms, both of which can be used in the same way.

One final important reminder: of all these remedies, only honey (and cloves in their natural form) are intended for consumption. All the others are to be gargled and spat out— don't swallow them!

CHAPTER 10:

TAME YOUR UNHEALTHY GUT WITH THESE PROVEN REMEDIES

Stop Bloating (and Look Thinner) in JUST ONE DAY!

We all want to look young and fit—so we exercise and watch what we eat.

But it still can take a bit of gymnastics to get those pants buttoned in the morning.

Problems like water retention and bloating can cause swelling everywhere from our bellies to our hands and our feet.

If you're tired of carrying around that excess gas or water weight, there is some really exciting news.

There are two powerful nutrients that can help you attack both bloating and water retention.

And you could see a difference in *as little as one day.*

The first powerhouse nutrient, believe it or not, is good ol' magnesium.

You've probably heard before how good magnesium is for your heart and even for anxiety.

But it actually attacks bloating in basically the same way.

Just like it causes your blood vessels to relax, it also relaxes the lining of your digestive tract. That can make it easier to clear up constipation or help you eliminate gas.

Around 200 mg. a day can help do the trick. Nature Made is a good source for magnesium citrate, the most easily absorbed form of the mineral. You can find the company on the Internet at **www.naturemade.com**.

The second natural cure is actually a weed you've probably been plucking out of your garden or striking down with the lawnmower for years.

It's the humble dandelion.

Dandelion acts as a natural diuretic, which means it can help you get rid of excess water you're retaining.

In a study on women published in the *Journal of Alternative and Complementary Medicine*, dandelion extract started working in JUST ONE DAY!

In fact, within just 5 hours, researchers noticed that patients were peeing in larger volumes and more frequently—a key indicator that they're eliminating retained fluids.

And the best part is that you don't have to start hunting through your backyard for this dandelion cure.

You can pick up dandelion extract as a supplement in liquid or capsule form for less than $10 a month. Just keep it in the medicine cabinet for the next time you feel like you're retaining water.

You can buy dandelion supplements affordably at **www.naturesway.com.**

Odd (but *Delicious*) Soup Seals Your Leaky Gut

It may be one of the most serious—and undiagnosed—health problems you're dealing with today.

And even when you can get a mainstream doctor to admit it's a real condition (and not just in your head), odds are he won't have a clue what to do about it.

This health menace is called Leaky Gut Syndrome, and millions of people may be suffering from it right now. With LGS, the lining of your intestinal tract fails, and toxins and waste leak into your body.

LGS can trigger serious inflammation and lead to health symptoms like:

- Bloating
- Digestive problems
- Fatigue
- Headaches
- Joint pain
- Skin blemishes, like acne
- And much, much more!

But, believe it or not, there's a tasty soup that alternative doctors are using right now to help seal leaky guts and bring people just like you back to health.

It's called bone broth, and it's a soup made from boiled bones, usually combined with herbs, spices, and other ingredients. The collagen from the bones can actually help seal our leaking guts and reduce the inflammation that causes lots of LGS symptoms.

So how can you make bone broth? Well, it's remarkably simple.

Any sort of bone can be used, though beef is the most popular choice. And while bone broth takes a long time to make, the results will be worth it.

Bone broth is also valuable because it can be made using leftover ingredients you might already have around. If you've been throwing away the bones of the meat you buy, making bone broth is a great way to put those bones to good use.

Again, preparing bone broth is a time-consuming process. But it's really not a lot of work—most of the time is spent letting the soup sit.

You'll need a few pounds (two or three, generally) of bone. If possible, make sure the bones come from a healthy, well-fed animal. While using bones leftover from other meals is a great way to be economical, you can also acquire bones specifically for bone broth from a local butcher or farmer.

There are many options for the non-bone ingredients in bone broth. Generally vegetables, spices, and herbs are added. A variety of combinations can be used, and experimentation can yield delicious results. Since it's hard to go seriously wrong don't be afraid to make a trial run.

An easy (and cheap) bone broth recipe

However, here is one fantastic recipe to start with: first get two pounds of beef bone with one onion, three medium-sized carrots, two stalks of celery, three tablespoons of vinegar, pepper, thyme, and kosher sea salt as the other ingredients.

Put the bones in a large pot and cover with water. Add the vinegar and let the concoction sit for a half hour. Then add the rest of the ingredients (after chopping the vegetables), and heat the soup to a boil. Then lower the heat to a simmer.

You'll have to let the soup simmer for the next 48 hours. Luckily, the dish will mostly take care of itself while you wait.

For the first few hours, remove any impurities that float to the top of the broth. Otherwise, you're free to accomplish whatever else is on your to-do list as the bone soup simmers on. After 48 hours have passed, remove the soup from heat and run it through a strainer, leaving only liquid.

Remember, this is just one possible recipe for bone broth. There are many possible variations. Most other types of bone will also take a shorter time to reach readiness. Chicken and other sorts of poultry will take 24 hours. Fish bones are ready after only 8 hours.

Bone broth can also be made in even larger bulk than the recipe above suggests. As long as you have a big enough pot, there is really no limit to the amount of the soup you can make. This can be a good way to efficiently prepare a dish that can last for many meals.

Bone broth, like any soup, can, of course, be eaten plain. This is a delicious option, but the dish can also be used as a base for stews, sauces, and even other soups. The versatility of bone broth is one of its major advantages.

Aside from gut-healing collagen, bone broth is filled with valuable minerals and amino acids. The long simmering process used to make bone broth extracts these nutrients. Bone broth contains large amounts of calcium and magnesium.

Better yet, bone broth is easy to digest. If a person has just caught or is recovering from a stomach bug, bone broth is a healthy meal that is unlikely to upset the digestive system.

You can easily make bone broth on your own, using the recipe here. If you want to buy bone broth, Bare Bones makes an organic, GMO-free variety.

You can check them out at **www.barebonesbroth.com**

Treat Your IBS Naturally with These 4 Drug-Free Breakthroughs

If you suffer from irritable bowel syndrome, you never know when a flare-up is going to happen.

A bout of diarrhea and abdominal pain can strike at any time, leaving you chained to the toilet and missing out on all your favorite activities.

But what if there was a way to say goodbye to your IBS symptoms without resorting to risky prescription drugs? Many patients have experienced IBS relief with these simple (and proven) alternative treatments.

IBS Breakthrough #1: Acupuncture

A traditional Chinese treatment, acupuncture helps with inflammation and is often used in combination with other treatments, such as herbal and probiotic supplements, to relieve IBS symptoms. Lots of patients report that their IBS is less severe when they undergo acupuncture regularly.

If you choose to give this treatment a try, make sure you go to a practitioner who has experience working specifically with

IBS patients. Go to **www.medicalacupuncture.org** to find a qualified acupuncturist near you.

IBS Breakthrough #2: Evening primrose oil

Many patients report that evening primrose oil supplements, when taken daily, reduce the frequency of their IBS symptoms. This natural herb is thought to calm the intestines and can also help regulate hormonal fluctuations that contribute to bowel irritability.

You can pick up NOW Foods Evening Primrose Oil at **www.pureformulas.com.**

IBS Breakthrough #3: Peppermint

The most common herbal remedy recommended for IBS, peppermint may be taken in several ways. If you choose to take the peppermint capsules that are sold by many health food stores, make sure you choose an enteric-coated variety. Non-enteric coated varieties sometimes lead to heartburn. Go to **www.naturesway.com** to find affordable peppermint supplements.

You can also try drinking 2–3 cups of peppermint tea each day. Brew your own peppermint tea by pouring 8 ounces of boiling water over 10–12 fresh peppermint leaves. Let the tea steep for 10 minutes, strain and enjoy.

IBS Breakthrough #4: Probiotic supplements

Some doctors believe that many cases of IBS are caused by an irregular balance of healthy probiotic bacteria in the intestines. If your IBS symptoms are due to such an imbalance, taking probiotic supplements (which are basically healthy gut bacteria) may prove highly effective in relieving them.

When choosing over-the-counter probiotic supplements,

look for ones that include proven bacterial strains like *L. acidophilus and B. infantis*. Store them carefully according to the package instructions so that you do not kill the live, active cultures.

Culturelle is a reputable supplier of quality probiotics, and you can find them online at **www.culturelle.com**.

Make sure you give any new treatment time to take effect before you decide whether it's effective for you. Different patients discover relief with different remedies, so don't give up until you find one that works.

Miracle Diet Soothes Even the Worst Gut Problems...So Why Haven't You Heard of It?

Sometimes the evidence of a serious gut problem won't be so obvious—like cramping, bloating, constipation, or diarrhea.

In fact, lots of times you may just feel sluggish, or have brain fog or difficulty concentrating.

When her own son was diagnosed with autism, Dr. Natasha Campbell-McBride developed an eating protocol called the GAPS (Gut and Psychology Syndrome or Gut and Physiology Syndrome) diet.

The goal was to produce a diet that could improve mental and emotional symptoms by healing the gut. And while the mainstream has been slow to catch on, so far the results have been astounding.

Since the gut and the brain are connected, everything that affects the gastrointestinal tract affects the brain. In addition, a dysfunctional gut leads to a variety of other health issues, including autoimmune disorders and inflammatory diseases.

Since the GAPS diet was reportedly successful in alleviating her son's autism symptoms, Dr. Campbell-McBride shared her discoveries with others. Since then, people of all ages who follow the GAPS diet continue to experience improvements in psychological issues and other diseases.

The goal of the GAPS protocol is to "heal and seal" the gut lining. There are many reasons why your gut lining becomes damaged. Diet, environmental toxins, and stress are a few examples of why these vital cells along the intestinal wall become damaged and destroyed.

A healthy gut is necessary for a healthy brain and body

The intestinal tract is lined with specialized cells that remove bacteria and other toxins as they help digest food. These cells live for about two or three days, then die off and are replaced with new cells.

Proteins, fats, enzymes, vitamins, and other molecules are needed for active and healthy cells to regenerate.

This network of cells, along with their death and reproduction, is managed by beneficial bacteria in the digestive system. Those who have gut problems—which can trigger psychological or emotional issues—are often lacking in the nutrients and beneficial bacteria that are necessary to produce healthy cells.

Animal studies show that when beneficial bacteria are removed, the gut lining and its processes are changed. When the cells reproduce, they are deformed and even sometimes cancerous.

Leaky gut triggers a dangerous autoimmune response

If you have a food allergy or intolerance, your digestive tract can become damaged. Undigested food particles travel through the damaged intestinal lining and into your bloodstream.

This condition, as we discussed earlier, is called Leaky Gut Syndrome, and is at the root of many autoimmune disorders.

The GAPS diet is effective because it heals holes in the intestinal lining where food and pathogens can pass through.

This treatment removes foods that damage the gut. That means you need to remove all grains, commercial dairy, starchy vegetables, and processed carbs.

It uses supplements like cod liver oil and probiotics, and fermented foods like kefir, sauerkraut, and miso to replenish beneficial bacteria. When fully healed, you are able to digest properly and eliminate food intolerances.

But you may need to detox first...

People who are overweight or who have severe health issues may need to start with a detoxification period. Raw fruits and vegetables are nature's internal cleansers, and a period of consuming only these detoxifying foods can boost the healing process.

After the cleansing period, whole, unprocessed animal foods and cooked vegetables should be reintroduced for nourishment. They're at the heart of the GAPS diet.

If you're interested in giving the GAPS diet a try, a great place to start is **www.gapsdiet.com**

Hidden Food Protein is Destroying Your Gut (and Your Health)

If you're suffering from gut problems—like gas, bloating, constipation, or diarrhea—there's a good chance these symptoms have been with you for years.

You may have even gone to the doctor's office, only to hear that all your tests came back negative...that they couldn't find anything.

But, believe it or not, there may be a very simple problem at the root of all your troubling gut issues.

You may be suffering from a gluten allergy or intolerance. It's hard to diagnose (and is often missed by doctors)—but once you fix it, you may see even your worst symptoms start to disappear, practically right away.

Gluten is a protein most commonly found in wheat products. And many health scientists believe it is the most common environmental trigger of autoimmune disease in the industrialized world.

Experts who study gluten believe that up to 60 percent of the population may suffer from some kind of bad reaction to gluten proteins.

When you have a serious gluten allergy, you may be diagnosed with celiac disease. But even if you don't have celiac disease, gluten proteins may spark an autoimmune response that can cause inflammation anywhere throughout your body.

Your body's response to gluten can wreck your health

We all learned in biology class a long time ago that our bodies produce antibodies in response to foreign invaders, like viruses. But when it comes to gluten, this process can work against you.

Toxic proteins in gluten, called gliadin, actually trigger the production of antibodies. And that's a big problem, because gliadin is similar in structure to several bodily tissues. So these antibodies mistakenly attack healthy tissue, unleashing intestinal damage and all sorts of other health problems.

An antibody test that measures certain anti-gliadin antibodies can be used. But many doctors don't bother, and the test isn't fool-proof by any means.

That's because other antibodies may be produced in response to gluten proteins, and they won't show up on the test.

An example of this is when you eat a certain food—for instance, wheat—and notice that you have a reaction to it. Maybe it causes you to become congested, get a migraine, or have joint pain.

You know that your body reacts a certain way to this substance, but food allergy tests may still produce negative results.

This doesn't mean that you are suffering any less than a person who tests positive for a food allergy, it just means that you are producing different antibodies. These antibodies, just like ones signaling celiac disease, attack healthy tissue anywhere in the body.

The tissue that gets attacked could be in your joints, thyroid, brain, or other areas. Even heart conditions, like myocarditis or cardiomyopathy, can be the result of a gluten sensitivity.

If you think you may be suffering from a gluten sensitivity, a good idea is to cut gluten from your diet and see if you notice any improvements. Lots of people notice their guts settling, their minds clearing, and their pain starting to disappear.

The Celiac Disease Foundation at **www.celiac.org** has a great list of foods that contain gluten.

The Thanksgiving Secret to Taming Ulcers

A prefect Thanksgiving feast takes a lot of preparation and work to pull off. So many dishes for just one meal.

But what if we told you one of these classic Thanksgiving staples could help ward off ulcers?

We know what you might be thinking— no way is corn-bread stuffing or mac and cheese going to help make my gut healthier.

You're right, they aren't.

It's actually the humble cranberry, rich in anti-inflammatory phytonutrients, antioxidants, and bacteria-fighting micronutrients, that is the king of the Thanksgiving spread.

And we're not talking about that gelatinous cran-log your sister slides out of a can and onto a plate every year.

We're talking about real cranberries. You know, the ones that are actually berry shaped, taste tart (like they naturally do), and don't require a can opener and a carving knife to serve or an insulin shot after eating.

Most of us are probably aware that cranberries are a tried-and-true remedy for urinary tract infections (UTI), but they have so much more to offer.

Cranberries contain proanthocyanidins (PACs). These are micronutrients that help fight UTIs. PACs do this by creating a barricade between bacteria and the lining of the urinary tract. But they also help fight other infections.

A study in the *Journal of Gastroenterology and Hepatology* found cranberries may protect the stomach from ulcers with the same mechanism.

By blocking bacteria, specifically *Helicobacter pylori*, from latching onto the stomach wall, PAC's inhibit their growth and reduce the risk of ulcers.

But, *H. pylori* doesn't just cause ulcers; it can infect them as well. Complications from these infections can lead to internal bleeding, stomach obstruction, and perforation (holes) of the stomach wall.

And if that wasn't enough—*H. pylori* infections increase the risk of stomach cancer.

Cranberries help your digestive tract in other ways too.

A study in *The FASEB Journal (published by the Federation of American Societies for Experimental Biology)* has shown cranberry may help to balance your gut bacteria. Drinking cranberry juice aids in the increase of *Bifidobacteria*, a gut-friendly microbe, while maintaining levels of other types of bacteria.

The more gut-friendly bacteria you have, the easier digestion should be for you.

In addition, its anti-inflammatory antioxidants help reduce the chances of gum disease by stopping cytokines. Cytokines send the message to our cells for an inflammatory response.

By halting cytokines, inflammation can be inhibited. Flavonoids and other antioxidants also help reduce risk of gum disease as well as colon cancer.

Cranberry also has heart protecting properties.

Inflammation, and oxidative stress can account for damage done to blood vessels and increase the risks of atherosclerosis (hardening of the arteries) and high cholesterol.

Simply drinking cranberry juice can decrease the triggering of enzymes involved in atherosclerosis and has been shown to reduce levels of LDL cholesterol (bad cholesterol) while also increasing levels of HDL cholesterol.

But that's not all cranberry can do for you.

In addition to halting oxidative stress and reducing inflammation (two major risk factors for cancer growth), studies on human cancer cells have shown cranberry to be a tumor repressor. By triggering programmed cell death it helps reduce tumor growth.

As a reminder, always choose organic cranberries, as the pesticides used in non-organic varieties can wreak havoc on your gut and overall health.

CHAPTER 11:

BANISH DIABETES WITH THESE *PROVEN* DRUG-FREE TREATMENTS

This Natural Salt Runs Circles Around Diabetes Meds

Maybe you retired years ago—but if you have diabetes, you've learned that managing it is practically a full-time job.

You're checking your blood sugar several times a day. You're watching what you eat and taking heavy-duty prescription drugs that have been linked to everything from diarrhea to bladder cancer.

Even worse? You've been told that you're going to be stuck on these diabetes meds for the rest of your life.

But what if NONE of that is true? Imagine being able to control your blood sugar without ever having to pop another pill again?

You'll never hear about this breakthrough from Big Pharma or even our government. But the fact is...

Scientists have discovered a natural remedy that BEATS diabetes meds

The news is being kept from millions of diabetics around the world right now. But you can get your hands on this amazing discovery for a lot less than what you might be spending on diabetes drugs now.

This miracle supplement is called berberine, and it's a salt that's found naturally in many types of fruits and vegetables and in an ancient Chinese herb called Coptis chinensis.

Berberine was actually first used by Chinese folk healers more than 5,000 years ago and can even be found in ancient Chinese medical texts. But recent research is now proving it may be the most powerful natural blood sugar control product to ever hit the market.

In fact, in an international study published in the medical journal *Metabolism*, **berberine ran circles around metformin**, one of the most popular diabetes drugs around.

Diabetics around the world have been choking down metformin for more than half a century, even though it's been linked to side effects like diarrhea, nausea, cramps, and vomiting.

Well, all that may be about to end.

In the 3-month trial, berberine performed just as well as metformin for lowering the key blood markers of diabetes (like A1c and fasting blood glucose).

Better still, berberine slashed fasting plasma insulin by a whopping 28 percent. And, again, that was after just 90 days! That means...

Better blood sugar in 3 months...
WITHOUT PRESCRIPTION DRUGS!

That's impressive enough—but berberine didn't stop there.

The patients who took berberine got an added benefit that wasn't seen in the metformin group. They also significantly lowered their "bad" cholesterol and triglycerides.

Keeping bad cholesterol and triglycerides in check is critical for your heart health—and lots of people with diabetes are also experiencing serious heart problems.

Berberine works by improving insulin resistance and activating a key enzyme in your body known as adenosine monophosphate-activated protein kinase, or AMPK. AMPK actually is responsible for controlling healthy metabolism in your body—kind of like a master switch.

By activating AMPK in your body, according to a report in the *Natural Medicine Journal*, berberine can have the same effect as exercise, dieting, and weight loss. That means...

Berberine is practically a diet in a pill!

And just like a diet, berberine can help you lose weight.

In one study of 37 people with metabolic syndrome—which can often lead to full-blown diabetes—patients who took 300 mg. of berberine three times a day for 3 months *dropped their body mass index by an impressive 13 percent!*

In fact, they lost enough weight to change their medical classification from obese to overweight! Berberine even helped reduce levels of stubborn belly fat.

And in another study out of South Dakota, published in a 2015 issue of *Phytomedicine*, people taking 500 mg. of berberine three times a day lost 5 pounds (or 3.6 percent of their body fat) in just 12 weeks.

Better blood sugar control, lower cholesterol AND weight loss? And berberine is delivering these results in months, not years.

It's no wonder research on berberine has been exploding over the past several years.

You don't have to be a doctor or a scientist to see that berberine is a blood sugar breakthrough—one that even outperformed metformin.

So why are the drug companies selling a fortune's worth of metformin, while many people have never heard of berberine?

It all comes down to money, of course. Berberine is a natural substance, so Big Pharma can't patent it. And if they could, you'd be hearing a lot more about it.

Plus, there's no army of drug sales reps visiting doctors' offices and pushing berberine.

Of course, if you're serious about controlling your blood sugar without prescription drugs (whether you have full diabetes yet or not), none of that should matter.

Berberine is now a fairly widely sold supplement, and you'll also see it as a key ingredient in many natural blood sugar formulations.

It's often combined with other natural substances that promote healthy blood sugar, like chromium.

Lose That Sweet Tooth *Forever* with This Mineral Trick

It's no big secret. When you're fighting diabetes, your biggest enemy is your sweet tooth.

It's hard to pass up that morning muffin or donut, or to skip dessert after a nice dinner out.

And holidays like Halloween and Christmas, with all the candy, cakes, and cookies everywhere? Well, they're just the worst.

Of course, mainstream medicine will tell you it's all a question of discipline. If you're serious about controlling your blood sugar, sacrifices need to be made.

But if you have out-of-control sugar cravings—and you could use a little extra help fighting them—chromium may just be the answer to your prayers.

Chromium is a natural mineral that alternative doctors have been using for years to help patients tame their sweet tooth. It's also found in varying levels in foods like lettuce, broccoli, onions, and green beans.

There is plenty of debate in the medical community about why it's so effective, but there are some things that we already know for sure.

First, chromium picolinate (the kind you typically see in supplements) has been found to help stabilize blood sugar and make insulin bind to cells to work more effectively. And, really, getting those wild blood sugar swings under control is critical to helping control sugar cravings.

One study found that people taking 600 mcg. of chromium picolinate for eight weeks seriously diminished their cravings for sweets and other carbohydrates.

Another study in the prestigious *Journal of the American College of Nutrition* found that chromium picolinate helped people with glucose tolerance issues in doses as low as 200 mcg. a day. People with more advanced diabetes or pre-diabetes will need larger doses.

Better still, research shows that chromium picolinate may help decrease weight gain and fat accumulation in people with type 2 diabetes. And weight control plays a big role in controlling both blood sugar and diabetes.

In fact, a study published in *Diabetes Care*, the journal of the American Diabetes Association, found that people taking chromium picolinate only gained less than half as much weight as patients who were treated with a placebo.

That's why many alternative doctors insist that chromium should be a major component of any natural diabetes treatment regimen. Better blood sugar control, less weight gain, and you might even lose your sweet tooth in the bargain.

What's not to love?

You can buy Nature's Bounty Mega Chromium Picolinate at **www.theonlinedrugstore.com.**

Turn Off Diabetic Nerve Pain with This Vitamin Fix

If you suffer from diabetes, you know there's a lot more involved than managing your blood sugar.

Diabetes comes with a laundry list of terrible side effects, including debilitating nerve pain, or neuropathy. The constant tingling, burning, and pain in your hands, feet, and legs can make life miserable.

Fortunately, the trick to making these nerve problems disappear may be easier than you ever imagined.

High blood sugar or diabetes can damage your nerves and cause neuropathy. For some folks, neuropathy is a minor annoyance—for others, it can be disabling.

Regardless of where you fall in this range, there's a natural substance that can help you combat this kind of nerve damage and the pain that comes with it—vitamin B12.

In fact, having low vitamin B12 levels can increase your risk of experiencing neuropathy, regardless if it's caused by diabetes or not.

But being diabetic puts you at even greater risk for experiencing neuropathy.

You see, diabetics are 22 percent more likely to be B12 deficient than folks without diabetes. And when you couple that with the fact that one of the leading diabetes medications, metformin, can rapidly decrease your vitamin B12 levels, you can see why many diabetics experience neuropathy.

So if you're diabetic and taking metformin, there's a good chance you'll develop neuropathy.

But diabetes and medications aren't your only worries when it comes to depleting B12 levels. Age, poor diet, certain acid-reflux meds and drinking alcohol can also lower your levels and lead to painful neuropathy.

On the other hand, maintaining a healthy B12 level can protect your nerves and help keep your neuropathy symptoms at bay.

Fortunately, upping your B12 intake is easy to do on your own. One easy way is to eat more B12-rich foods, like red meat, eggs and poultry.

Or you can simply take a B12 supplement. For best results, find a supplement that contains B12 in its natural form, methylcobalamin.

Bio-Active B-12 from Gold Leaf Nutritionals (which is affiliated with the Alliance for Advanced Health) is a product that is easily absorbed by your body.

You can get it at **www.goldleafnutritionals.com**

If you suspect you're B12 deficient, you can also talk to your doctor and get a simple blood test.

Diabetes Breakthrough Works in 1 DAY!

If you have diabetes (or are on your way to getting it), you've probably been told how risky it is for your health.

And you've probably tried everything from finger pricks to pricey pills to painful insulin injections to keep your blood sugar numbers in line.

But it looks like controlling your blood sugar may have just gotten A LOT easier.

Recent research has revealed a foolproof way of eating that can help you lower your blood sugar fast.

And the best part? You may see results in as little as one day.

The secret formula is eating three low-carb meals a day. That's it.

Researchers from the University of Michigan split 32 postmenopausal women with healthy blood sugar into four different groups.

They were all given meals with different amounts of carbs (from 30–60 percent of the total calories). All meals had the same calorie counts.

After eating the meals, all of the groups were measured for

insulin resistance, a major contributor to high blood sugar, diabetes and fatty liver disease.

The low-carb groups showed *significantly* lower levels of insulin resistance when compared with the high-carb groups.

And it took only three meals—as in just ONE day of eating.

However, the high-carb groups had consistently high levels of insulin resistance. That remained true even in the high-carb groups that exercised regularly, which is supposed to lower insulin resistance and blood sugar levels.

So what's the lesson here? You can better control your blood sugar and lower your risk of developing diabetes in just 24 hours by cutting carbs.

And the good news for low-carb diets doesn't end there.

Another recent study shows that diabetics who ate diets that were 40 percent carbs or lower can slash their liver fat nearly in half in six weeks. If liver fat is left untreated, it contributes to diabetes and liver cirrhosis.

Simply put, cutting your carbs to around 30 percent may keep you from the enduring a lifelong struggle with one of America's biggest killers.

Don't worry, though: Giving up carbs doesn't mean you're also giving up flavor.

Instead, it gives you the green light to enjoy breakfasts full of eggs and bacon, chicken Caesar salad lunches and steak and green bean dinners. Just be sure to pass on the carb-heavy dessert.

Wartime Coffee Substitute Fights Diabetes *and* Arthritis

Many folks can't think of anything worse than a morning without coffee.

And coffee is jam-packed with powerful compounds that can thwart off ailments like cancer, Alzheimer's and heart issues.

But there's another morning brew that could boost your health and even protect you from diabetes and arthritis.

It's a powerful root that's been used as a coffee replacement and additive for centuries and is now being recognized for its potent health-boosting powers.

It's called chicory, the root of a blue flowering plant, and it's been making its way into America's coffee cups since the 1800s.

You see, when the city of New Orleans was under siege during the American Civil War, coffee supplies dwindled to near nothing. However, inventive locals stretched out their coffee supplies by adding roasted chicory root.

While it lacks caffeine, chicory root is cheap and tasty and makes a great addition to coffee. So even after the supply lines were reopened, citizens of New Orleans kept chicory in their coffee. In fact, chicory coffee is still available in many New Orleans restaurants.

But what folks didn't realize at the time was that adding this earthy root to their coffee wasn't just padding the supply. It was also boosting their health.

In more recent years, chicory root has been the subject of many health studies. It's been shown to reduce inflammation, delay or prevent the onset of diabetes, and even help folks' arthritis.

In one study, folks who took chicory root extract saw improved A1c levels, which is an indicator of diabetes. In addition, researchers found that chicory also significantly improved adiponectin levels. Adiponectin is a protein that's involved in regulating glucose levels.

Both of these findings showed that enjoying chicory regularly could thwart the development and/or onset of diabetes.

Another study found that chicory root also improves arthritis symptoms. A clinical trial done by the Rheumatic Diseases Division at the University of Texas Southwestern Medical Center's Department of Internal Medicine shows that chicory root may also be able to combat the painful symptoms of arthritis.

When people aged 50 or older who had osteoarthritis of the hip or knee took chicory, some showed a 20 percent improvement in pain and stiffness. This means chicory root might help reduce the pain and stiffness caused by arthritis.

Perhaps of all these incredible abilities, reducing inflammation is the key to chicory's powers, since it's full of plant polyphenols that can stomp out inflammation and curtail its effects on the body. This is so important because inflammation is considered the gateway to many chronic diseases.

Chicory is easy to get. You can look for it in health food store or online retailer websites.

In addition, there are a few coffee makers that offer coffee and chicory blends. The most popular is Cafe Du Monde, and their coffees are available through their website, **CafeDuMonde.com**

The Blood Sugar Bomb Hiding in Your Water Bottle

We've all gotten an earful over the years about all the different ways that food can give us diabetes.

They tell us to cut out the bread...the pasta...the soda... fructose...and all our favorite desserts.

But what many people don't realize is that one of our biggest diabetes risks might not be coming from food itself.

It's coming from the packaging our food arrives in.

There's a chemical called bisphenol-A (BPA) that's being used in plastic water bottles, soup cans, and countless other food packaging today. And if you're not careful, it could put you on the fast-track to diabetes.

BPA is used as a plastic hardener—but there are plenty of others things it does, too. For example, it's an endocrine disruptor, which means it wreaks havoc on your body's hormone levels.

Scientists started uncovering the risk more than a decade ago, when they learned that BPA exposure could trigger insulin resistance in mice. In fact, it was causing the exact same insulin problems we usually see in someone who is starting to develop diabetes.

And the news just kept getting worse from there.

In fact, a study out of Spain in 2012 found that BPA can trick your body into releasing TWICE as much insulin as you need. The next thing you know, you're dealing with blood sugar swings that are wildly out of control.

Now, if you go to the supermarket today, you'll see lots of packaged foods and beverages that are claiming to be "BPA-Free." But that doesn't mean we're out of the woods.

It's still used in the linings of many canned foods. That means you're always better off buying fresh vegetables and making your own homemade soup.

BPA is also found in packaging for many frozen meals, which are often loaded with lots of unhealthy preservatives anyway.

You're also much better off avoiding using plastic dishes in the microwave. Many have BPA, and the heat can make it leach into your food. Go with your regular ceramic dishes instead.

And, finally, don't use any water bottles unless they're BPA-Free. If you have older water bottles around the house and aren't sure, make an investment in some new ones.

Finally, if your grandkids are using older "hand me down" bottles and sippy cups, they may have BPA and it's a wise idea to replace them.

Delicious (and Forbidden) Treat CRUSHES Insulin Resistance

If you're diabetic, you've probably been told dessert is an indulgence of the past.

Well real dessert, at any rate…you've still got the green light on sugar-free gelatin and tasteless baked goods chock-full of chemical sweeteners.

Who wants those anyway?

But as it turns out, lime Jell-O and Splenda-filled macaroons aren't your only options.

Researchers have discovered there's a decadent and delicious dessert snack that helps fight diabetes at its core.

This powerful food is chocolate (and I mean REAL chocolate, not the sugar-loaded stuff in the candy aisle).

And because chocolate's antioxidant levels are off the charts, it's long been the subject of many health studies.

More recently, a study published in the *British Journal of Nutrition* discovered that chocolate can defend your body against two of the biggest risk factors for diabetes—insulin resistance and elevated liver enzymes.

For the study, researchers analyzed the chocolate consumption habits of around 1,200 people who were enrolled in a heart health study.

The aim of the study was to determine whether eating chocolate had an effect on insulin resistance, a condition that messes with your blood sugar and increases your risk of Type 2 diabetes and heart disease.

In addition, the researchers looked at what chocolate can do to your liver enzymes. Abnormal levels of liver enzymes are also a key driver of Type 2 diabetes.

Turns out that 81.8 percent of the subjects ate chocolate at a rate of 24.8 grams a day.

When they compared the chocolate eaters' health stats to those of the nonchocolate-eating group…they were SHOCKED!

It turns out the chocolate eaters not only saw reduced insulin resistance; they also experienced an improvement in their liver enzymes.

But what was even more incredible…these results remained true even when they factored for age, sex, diet, education and lifestyle.

Now, 24.8 grams is about a fourth of an average-sized chocolate bar. This means eating just a tiny bit of chocolate a day can keep diabetes at bay!

And the good news keeps coming…

Another study found that folks who ate 100 grams of chocolate (an average-sized chocolate bar) a day lowered their risk of heart disease by 11 percent and lowered their risk of dying from heart issues by 25 percent.

While this is great news of anyone looking to ditch diabetic desserts, keep in mind not all chocolate is good for diabetics. Ultra-processed and extra-sugary varieties probably won't help you fight diabetes.

Instead, look for organic chocolate varieties that have a

cocoa content of 70 percent or more (which you can now find at most grocery stores). This way, you can enjoy a real dessert and fight diabetes at the same time.

Cover-Up! Top-Selling Drug is *Giving You Diabetes*

It may be one of the greatest cover-ups in modern medicine… and it's one that could threaten your life or the life of someone you love.

You can't turn on the television these days without seeing a commercial for a so-called cholesterol-lowering statin drug like Lipitor or Zocor. These medications are being handed out like Halloween candy and have made the drug companies billions.

But statins come with a dark secret that's being kept from millions of patients like you. They could send your risk of potentially deadly diabetes through the roof!

You see, statins were first discovered in the 1970s…and once they hit the market, we were bombarded by health messages about how bad cholesterol is for us. Coincidental timing, right?

Statins are supposed to lower your levels of LDL or "bad" cholesterol, to reduce your chances of heart attack or stroke. Never mind that studies have proven that they hardly extend lives at all, and come with serious side effects like cataracts and muscle pain.

And now we know that statins may put you on a dangerous

path to type 2 diabetes.

You see, when statins first hit the market, scientists still didn't fully understand how they work in your body. Now we have evidence that taking statin drugs can boost blood sugar levels and lead to the development of type 2 diabetes.

A study in Finland followed a number of male subjects between the ages of 45 and 70, tracking their blood glucose levels over time. Individuals who were taking statin drugs were a whopping 46 percent more likely to develop type-2 diabetes than those who did not take the drugs.

This wasn't a one-time thing, either...studies since have also proven the link between statins and diabetes.

And, again, this isn't the only problem you get with statins. The side effects include muscle pain, cataracts, liver impairment, sinus problems and other effects that can be so serious that many people have stopped taking the drugs.

Lucky them, right?

The fact is, statins are the most over-prescribed medications around today, especially given that there's scant evidence that they extend lives.

If you're taking a statin drug right now (they're even being given to people in nursing homes!) your best bet is to talk to your doctor about whether you really need to be on them.

And if he insists, do yourself a favor and get a second opinion.

This "Apple Pie Remedy" Lowers Blood Sugar and Cholesterol

When it comes to the best smells ever created, cinnamon is awfully hard to beat. There's nothing like the scent of cinnamon wafting through the house from a fresh-baked apple pie.

But cinnamon can do a lot more than make our taste buds happy. In fact, it may be one of the most powerful underground diabetes fighters around.

And adding cinnamon to your supplement regimen may be the secret to enjoying your best blood sugar control in years.

Research has now proven that cinnamon lowers blood sugar, triglyceride, and cholesterol levels in people who suffer from type 2 diabetes.

In one landmark study, researchers saw results after just 40 days of putting people on cinnamon. Cinnamon was so effective at reducing high blood sugar that for some people the results continued even two weeks after the study ended!

Cinnamon seems to work by lowering insulin resistance, which is a key marker for diabetes.

In another study out of Pakistan, people who took cinnamon experienced significant reductions in LDL or "bad" cholesterol, while their HDL or "good" cholesterol wasn't affected.

Sixty diabetic patients with an average age of 52 participated in the research. One group received placebo capsules filled with wheat flour. Other participants received either 1 gram, 3 grams, or 6 grams of cassia cinnamon each day for 40 days while eating normal diets.

Cassia cinnamon can be easily purchased at most grocery stores for use in baking.

Researchers drew blood from the participants after 20, 40, and 60 days. They found fasting glucose levels fell between 18–29 percent in patients using cinnamon (that could be enough to bring your blood sugar out of the diabetic zone).

Triglyceride levels dropped 23–30 percent during the testing period, and when total cholesterol was measured, scientists discovered levels decreased 12–26 percent in groups taking cinnamon capsules.

LDL cholesterol dropped an impressive 7–27 percent, and the most significant reductions were in people taking 3 and 6 grams of cinnamon a day.

And even better? Some patients continued to register similar decreases in blood sugar and cholesterol levels up to 20 days after they stopped ingesting cinnamon.

Cinnamon contains no calories and can be added to your diet inexpensively. In addition to its effects on glucose, triglycerides, and cholesterol, cinnamon is a powerful antioxidant that can fight oxidative stress.

You can add cinnamon easily to oatmeal or even coffee. Your best bet may be to take cinnamon supplements. Puritan's Pride sells an affordable cinnamon supplement at **www.puritan.com**.

Beat Diabetes (and Other Nagging Health Problems) with This Kitchen Staple

You might not know it, but you probably have a multi-purpose health product sitting in your kitchen cupboard right now.

And it may be able to deliver blood sugar numbers that will have your doctor picking his jaw up off the floor!

It's simply apple cider vinegar, and it's been renowned as a folk remedy for thousands of years. Now, health researchers are proving that it could be the secret to better blood sugar control and helping countless health problems vanish!

Studies have proven that apple cider vinegar has potent antiglycemic effects, which means it helps keep your blood sugar at healthy levels.

High blood sugar is bad news for a number of reasons: it's most commonly associated with type 2 diabetes, and it's also linked with damage to the organs, immune system, and cardiovascular system.

Apple cider vinegar blocks some of your digestion of starch, which is one of the most common culprits of blood sugar spikes. It also improves your insulin sensitivity, which is a key marker for diabetes.

And that's not all apple cider vinegar can do. Here are 6 more reasons you'll want to start incorporating this kitchen cure into your daily routine.

#1: Eases upset stomach and promotes digestion

If you're feeling queasy or having digestive problems, sip some apple cider vinegar diluted in water—it has powerful antibiotic effects that can help clear up any bacterial infection that's plaguing your digestive system.

It improves your general gut health, too. Because apple cider vinegar inhibits your body's digestion of starch, it frees up those starches to feed the friendly bacteria in your gut. This comes with the side benefit of strengthening your immune system as well.

#2: Helps you lose weight

Apple cider vinegar may help with weight loss. Apple cider vinegar contains acetic acid, which can give your metabolism a boost and reduce appetite (which is a big help for diabetics).

And, again, by blocking some digestion of starch, apple cider vinegar prevents your body from absorbing those calories.

#3: Prevents heartburn

Sipping apple cider vinegar to prevent heartburn might seem counterintuitive, but most of the time, heartburn is actually caused by not having enough acid in the stomach. Apple cider vinegar gives you some relief by bringing your stomach acid levels back up to normal.

#4: Helps with sore throat

Apple cider vinegar is a great germ-killer. When you feel a sore throat coming on, gargle with equal parts apple cider vinegar and warm water to clear out the infection.

#5: Soothes congestion

Next time you find yourself stuffed up with a cold, reach for your apple cider vinegar along with your tissues. Besides its germ-killing properties, apple cider vinegar contains potassium, which thins mucus and helps you breathe better.

#6: Makes hair shiny and prevents dandruff

Apple cider vinegar is a great natural treatment for your hair and scalp. Dilute ¼ cup of apple cider vinegar in 2 cups of water, pour over your hair, and then rinse with cold water.

The vinegar removes any product buildup in your hair and leaves it soft and shiny. If you have dandruff, spritz a mixture of equal parts apple cider vinegar and water on your scalp, wrap your head in a towel, and leave it in for up to an hour before washing it out.

So how do you go about drinking apple cider vinegar? Well, don't just swig from the bottle.

Pure apple cider vinegar is very strong, so when you consume it, be sure to dilute it with water or juice first.

GNC also makes a line of apple cider vinegar supplements. You can buy them at your local store, or check out **www.gnc.com.**

Miracle "Jesus Oil" Tackles Cancer, Diabetes and MORE

It's one of the most memorable stories from the Holy Bible.

God handed down to Moses the formula for a Holy Anointing Oil—one that became a key part of both Jewish and Christian tradition.

Even Jesus Christ Himself was anointed with the oil, and was said to use it in his healing miracles.

Now, 2,000 years after the death of Jesus, this powerful oil is still performing miracles for people with hopeless cases of cancer, diabetes, and even learning disorders.

And stunned scientists are starting to admit that…

The "Jesus Oil" may be the greatest natural healing compound on Earth!

In fact, a key ingredient in this holy oil is becoming a major medical breakthrough.

In the Bible, you'll see that one of the components of the holy anointing oil is something called kaneh-bosom. Now, researchers have discovered that kaneh-bosom is actually a type of cannabis extract.

Of course, this is where things get controversial. When

many people hear of cannabis, they make a natural connection to marijuana.

But the fact is, cannabis extract has been an important natural healing compound for thousands of years.

"There can be little doubt about a role for cannabis in Judaic religion," said Carl Ruck, professor of classical mythology at Boston University.

And there's little doubt that high-potency cannabis oil is becoming one of the most important healing substances ever, capable of wiping away some of the worst diseases of aging.

Just ask Paul Hanson, a 65-year-old man who had been struggling with type 2 diabetes.

In August 2011, Paul weighed 215 pounds...and had a blood sugar level of 12%.

He began treating his condition with high-potency cannabis oil...and after just 7 weeks, his blood sugar levels dropped by an astounding 62%... back to NORMAL levels!

According to Paul, *"My diabetes is gone! I continue to keep doing a small dose of the oil...and today the scale said 162.5 pounds. **I did not change my diet, but the oil did it for me.**"*

Even more incredible, Paul explained that, *"I was diagnosed with dyslexia as a kid. I could never spell...but for some reason I can spell 10-times better now!!"*

So what's the secret?

Well, in 1990, an organic chemist and professor of medicinal chemistry at the Hebrew University of Jerusalem—not too far from where Jesus performed HIS miracles—made one of the greatest medical discoveries of the 20th century.

His name is Dr. Raphael Mechoulam...and he identified a previously unknown regulatory system found throughout the entire human body.

It's a God-given, **built-in** mechanism specifically designed to cure disease.

That's right—your body is **already** wired to shut down

nearly ALL diseases...

It's called the Endocannabinoid System (or the ECS.)

To put this discovery into context, retired cardiac heart surgeon Dr. David Allen said during a recent interview that:

"The discovery of the ECS is the single most important medical discovery EVER."

"More people will be saved by manipulation of the ECS than are currently saved by surgery...and I'm a heart surgeon saying this."

It "performs some miraculous functions in the body... we're finding out now that it controls diabetes...it controls cancer...it controls whether or NOT you can survive a heart attack or stroke."

This is a system that God placed in every single human being on the planet (as well as almost all of God's creatures) as a way to naturally ward off disease.

And—as Dr. Mechoulam first discovered—high-potency cannabis oil contains over 480 natural compounds that provide the KEY to "turning-on" your body's own Endocannabinoid System!

So what happens when you use high-potency cannabis oil to turn on your body's natural healing system?

Just ask Connie.

In 2011, Connie was diagnosed with life-threatening cancer (the same cancer that took Farrah Fawcett's life). She was given 4...maybe 6 months to live.

Not only that, but Connie also suffered debilitating pain from a previous heart surgery AND had two spots of skin cancer on her collar bone.

Incredibly, she rejected traditional treatments like radiation and chemotherapy and turned to high-potency cannabis oil after hearing about it through her caregiver.

Within 48-hours, the oil worked to completely remove the skin cancer…then, after another two weeks, the pain in her sternum, as well as the nerve pain she'd suffered through had become "almost non-existent."

And then she learned that—even though she *never* received chemotherapy or radiation—her cancer was completely gone!

Research is also showing that high-potency cannabis oil holds promise as a treatment for heart problems, seizures, and many other diseases that had once seemed hopeless.

It's truly a miracle!

And high-potency cannabis oil is truly versatile. It can be taken orally or even as a suppository. While it does contain THC, the same psychoactive compound from marijuana, taking the oil as a suppository can erase any of THC's unwanted effects.

Another option is to try cannabidoil (often known as CBD oil). It's milder, while still effective in treating a variety of health conditions.

Of course, getting your hands on cannabis oil is where things can get a little trickier. There are plenty of cannabis oils sold online, but they often lack enough potency and having them shipped to you may be illegal.

Your best bet is to get high-potency cannabis oil from a state that has legalized medical cannabis. It's illegal to transport marijuana or cannabis oil across state lines. So, depending on your condition, you may want to consider relocating.

The 29 states where it is now legalized include Alaska, Arizona, Arkansas, California, Colorado, Connecticut, Delaware, Florida, Hawaii   , Illinois, Maine, Maryland, Massachusetts, Michigan, Minnesota, Montana, Nevada, New Hampshire, New Jersey, New Mexico, New York, North Dakota, Ohio, Oregon, Pennsylvania, Rhode Island, Vermont, Washington, Washington, DC, and West Virginia.

Laws vary in each state and in Washington, DC. But, in general, you'll need to get a medical marijuana card. That typically requires proof of residence, a qualifying condition (such as cancer, glaucoma, or multiple sclerosis) and a doctor to sign your forms.

You can find a doctor who may be willing to help at **www.marijuanadoctors.com**.

BLAST AWAY STUBBORN POUNDS WITH THESE WEIGHT-LOSS SECRETS

The "Voodoo Secret' to Stopping Hunger Attacks

We all start our diets with the best of intentions.

But if you're someone who is constantly hungry...if it's hard to go an hour or two without reaching for the chips or cookies...dieting can be a lost cause.

Luckily, there's an amazing Asian secret that can help you control your hunger pangs and start peeling off the pounds. But, believe it or not, most American mainstream doctors have never even heard of it!

It's called konjac, and it comes from an Asian plant known as "voodoo lilly."

But there's no voodoo magic when it comes to how konjac helps you lose weight—just lots of science and common sense.

You see, konjac is a soluble fiber that comes from the root of the voodoo lilly, and it's often added to foods under the name "glucomannan" to help people feel more full.

But now you can also get konjac as a tablet, capsule or powder (we'll show you how in a second) to help get your hunger under control.

Konjac is an incredibly effective appetite suppressant. Just taking the product with at least 8 ounces of liquid prior to each meal will help you feel full on much less food.

But, believe it or not, that's not all konjac can do.

Konjac also has been shown to improve blood sugar levels. Because it slows the process of food emptying from your stomach, konjac can help even out blood sugar levels after meals and reduce insulin spikes.

This can help dieters avoid post-meal energy slumps that can leave you craving sweets and other junk food.

Finally, there are indications that konjac helps reduce LDL cholesterol and triglyceride levels. A small study on healthy men showed reductions in LDL, triglycerides and systolic blood pressure *after just four weeks.*

And here's the best part—the guys in the study made no other changes to their diets or activity levels.

Konjac appears to block the transport of cholesterol from the liver into the bloodstream. It also may increase the activity of 7-alpha hydroxylase, an enzyme that helps convert cholesterol into bile acids.

There are a few things you'll want to consider before adding konjac to your supplement regimen.

First, remember, konjac is like any other fiber—you don't want to overdo it, or you could end up with problems like diarrhea, gas, or bloating. So always follow the manufacturer's instructions.

And because konjac slows the entry of glucose into your bloodstream, it may not be right for you if you're taking insulin or other diabetic medications.

Finally, you can buy konjac as a tablet, capsule, or powder. But you can't always guarantee that the capsule will open in your stomach where you want it (as opposed to your throat or intestines).

So the best way to take konjac is as a powder. You can buy konjac powder at **www.konjacfoods.com.**

Warning! Mainstream HIDING Weight-Loss Surgery Deaths

It's become the latest surgical fad, turning doctors into millionaires.

Every year, thousands of overweight people are being lured into risky gastric bypass weight-loss surgery.

Mainstream surgeons will tell you that the operation—which reduces your stomach to about the size of an egg—will literally melt the pounds away. They'll tell you it can cure diabetes and maybe even save your life.

But there's a dark secret about gastric bypass that many patients aren't being told about. It's already killed people in every part of the world.

It's a problem that NOBODY is talking about. And if you're not careful, you or someone you love could be next.

In fact, that's a lesson that the family of Angela Jones learned the hard way. The British mother lost more than 300 pounds in a year after getting gastric bypass.

But the problem was that she couldn't STOP losing weight. Her weight plummeted to less than 60 pounds and she had to have a feeding tube inserted.

Her health continued to deteriorate, and Angela was dead just a few years after her surgery.

And, believe it or not, Angela was not alone. Malnutrition and problems absorbing nutrients are common after gastric bypass, and many people find their bodies are literally starving.

One 9-year study of people from Pennsylvania uncovered 440 deaths and found that the 5-year death rate after gastric bypass was an unacceptable 6 percent.

They never mention that in the marketing literature, do they?

And even people who survive gastric bypass may find themselves tackling another problem—drug or alcohol addiction. That's because they may replace their food addictions with other vices instead.

That's called "addiction transfer." In fact, a study out of New York looked at 150 people who'd gotten gastric bypass and found significant increases in drug and alcohol dependency after the surgeries.

So why does the mainstream keep promoting this potentially dangerous operation? It's all about the money.

The average cost of gastric bypass is $23,000, and mainstream surgeons aren't about to turn their backs on that kind of cash.

But the evidence is mounting that gastric bypass can create more (and more serious) problems than it solves.

If you or someone you love is looking to lose weight, skipping this surgery just might save your life. Instead, use the scientifically proven strategies in this book to quickly and safely lose those extra pounds.

TORCH Fat with This "Banned" Berry

Are you tired of feeling heavy and sluggish?

Do you wish you could put your clothes on and feel confident about the way you look in them?

Or ever taken a look in the mirror and realized you're carrying a spare tire around your waist?

The thing is, you're not alone.

So many of us have struggled with weight gain, and it gets harder and harder to keep those pounds off as we age.

Fortunately, there's now an incredible (and tasty) way to keep your weight in check.

A groundbreaking study shows that a "banned" berry may hold the secret to helping you win the war against flab for good.

The berry is from the mulberry tree, and it contains a powerful compound called rutin.

Rutin has been the subject of many weight loss studies because it can "activate" brown fat. Unlike white fat, which is stored by the body to later be used as energy (and also makes you gain weight), brown fat's sole purpose is to keep your body warm.

You see, brown fat is like an internal torch—it burns obesity-causing white fat and makes heat in the body. Because of this, folks who have more brown fat typically carry less excess weight than those who have less brown fat.

Exposure to cold temperature was once thought to be the only way to activate brown fat, but now researchers have discovered that rutin can also kick your brown fat into gear.

To prove this, scientists tested rutin in obese rats.

For this study, researchers from China used both genetically obese mice and mice with diet-induced obesity. Both sets of mice were given supplemental rutin in their drinking water and fed the same diet.

At the end of the experiment, the scientists found that the mice from both groups had increased energy, improved blood sugar and lost weight. This was because the rutin "activated" the mice's brown fat.

There's just one problem...Mulberry is banned in several cities.

Well, in tree form, anyway...

Many cities, like El Paso and Albuquerque, have outlawed the planting of mulberry trees, due to their intense pollen output.

Fortunately, though, you can still legally get your hands on mulberry extract and rutin supplements, regardless of where you live, in natural health stores and through online retailers like Amazon.com.

One study suggests 425 mg. of rutin daily for weight loss.

Puritan's Pride makes a 500 mg. rutin supplement you can pick up at **www.puritan.com.**

Canadian Swamp Seed CURED Metabolic Syndrome

If you're carrying some extra weight around your belly, you know that it's more than a cosmetic problem.

It's a genuine threat to your health…and, long term, even your life.

In fact, if you have excess weight around your midsection, high triglycerides, and elevated blood sugar, you may have developed a condition known as metabolic syndrome.

That means you're at serious risk for developing full-blown type 2 diabetes, heart disease, and other serious medical issues.

Fortunately, if you have metabolic syndrome, there's still time to turn the situation around and reclaim your health.

And the cure may be a simple seed found in some of the nastiest places around, including Canadian swamps!

This amazing metabolic syndrome breakthrough is flaxseed—and it's turning out to be a more powerful disease-fighter than the medical community ever realized.

Flaxseeds are an excellent source of fiber and those heart-healthy omega-3 fatty acids (like the kind you get in fish oil). And alternative doctors have been recommending flaxseed for years to help lower cholesterol.

But flaxseed is also a key weapon in the war against metabolic syndrome.

In one study out of the Middle East, researchers divided adults with metabolic syndrome into two groups—one group got just lifestyle advice, and the other got the advice plus 30 g. a day of flaxseed.

More than 80 percent of the folks who added flaxseed to their diet got rid of their metabolic syndrome completely.

They were completely cured.

They lost more weight, shrunk their waistlines, and even reduced their insulin resistance, a key marker for diabetes.

Better still, flaxseed is dirt cheap. You can pick up a bag for less than $10 (look for the ground varieties, or grind it yourself), and you can incorporate flaxseed into lots of recipes, like muffins or other baked goods.

Spectrum Essentials makes an organic, ground flaxseed you can pick up at **www.vitacost.com.**

The easiest way to get more flaxseed is to add it to oatmeal, yogurt, or smoothies. You can store it in your freezer and it practically lasts forever. You're more likely to run out of it than see it go bad.

Flaxseed will add a little bit of a nutty taste, which most people enjoy.

This Diet FORCES Your Body to Lose Weight (But is it Right For You?)

There is no shortage of diets on the market promising to help you lose weight. And when you go looking for advice, it can get confusing really quickly.

One doctor will tell you to go low-fat...and another will recommend low-carb...and there are even fad diets telling you to eat nothing but cabbage soup!

Who wants to live like that anyway?

But there's one diet that's guaranteed to activate your body's natural fat-burning processes.

And the best part? You get to load up on your favorite "forbidden" foods like T-bone steaks and scrambled eggs.

It's the ketogenic diet, and it's a variation of low-carb dieting that leans heavily toward the "no-carb" end of the spectrum. But because the ketogenic diet emphasizes foods high in healthy fats, you'll feel fuller longer with less food.

The goal of a ketogenic diet plan is to trigger a process called "ketosis," where you burn your body's fat stores instead of sugar for fuel (more on that in a moment).

The ketogenic diet consists of mostly fat—think avocadoes, cheese, bacon, and real butter. On this diet, you will also eat a moderate amount of protein like chicken, beef, fish, and eggs.

The only restriction is the amount of carbohydrates you will eat—no sugar, rice, pasta, or bread.

Sending your body into ketosis

In order to understand what ketosis is and how to use it to your advantage, it helps to understand a bit about how your body metabolizes fuel.

You see, most people follow a diet that is fairly high in carbohydrates. As such, the human body utilizes these carbs by breaking them down into glucose and converting them to fuel.

In the absence of carbohydrates, the body turns to stored fat for fuel. Ketones (where the ketogenic diet gets its name from) are one of the products produced by the liver as a result of fat metabolism.

On the ketogenic diet, a person restricts carbohydrate intake significantly, forcing the body into ketosis. For most people, the result is fat loss with very little loss of muscle tissue. Another draw is that you can get good results without strenuous exercise.

Upon starting the ketogenic diet, of course the initial goal is to get into ketosis—the state in which the body burns fat for fuel.

To accomplish this goal, the standard ketogenic diet calls for restricting carbs to 20–30 grams a day. Most experts agree that this carb-restricted regimen should be followed for the first week. This period of time is the most difficult part of the diet.

During the initial phase, you do NOT count calories (sounds good, right?) and you eat fat until you're satisfied.

After a day or two, many people find that they are less

hungry because cravings for sugar and other carbs are either greatly diminished or eliminated altogether.

After about 3 to 5 days, the average person is in ketosis and well on their way to reaching their weight-loss goals. After the first week, carbohydrate amounts can be increased slightly.

Delicious ketogenic food choices

On the ketogenic diet, there are many delicious food that you can eat. It is much more important to consider what you are eating as opposed to how much.

A big part of the ketogenic diet is meat, vegetables, and eggs. Dairy is also allowed, but read labels to make sure there aren't added sugars.

A typical breakfast on the ketogenic diet consists of as many eggs as you want, breakfast meat like bacon, sausage, or ham, and black coffee or tea.

Lunch suggestions include a hamburger without the bun and a side salad with full fat salad dressing. Read the labels on salad dressing, though. Many commercial dressings add significant amounts of sugar.

A keto-worthy dinner might include steak or fish with a side of steamed broccoli or asparagus with cheese or real butter.

Again, this diet encourages you to eat until you are full. Not being hungry is a big part of what makes this diet doable.

The ketogenic diet has been touted as one of the quickest ways to lose weight. Those on the ketogenic diet usually lose more water weight initially than those on other diets—up to *10 pounds in the first two weeks.*

After that, most people continue to experience losses of 2–4 pounds of fat per week.

Dieters who turn to the ketogenic diet tend to be people who are severely overweight or people with health problems related to sugar and carb addictions.

Others who may not necessarily be overweight but would like to boost energy levels may also benefit from the ketogenic lifestyle diet.

A great resource for ketogenic-friendly meals is "The Keto-genic Cookbook," which you can buy at **www.amazon.com.**

6 Common Drugs That Are BLOCKING Your Weight Loss

You're exercising like a Navy SEAL. You're barely eating enough to keep a rabbit alive.

And the scale still won't budge!

If you're finding that you can't lose weight…no matter what you try…there's a dirty secret you'll probably never hear about at your doctor's office.

There are entire classes of prescription drugs—medications that are making Big Pharma BILLIONS—that may actually be blocking you from losing weight.

And until you work with your doctor to get these medications out of your life, or find less risky alternatives, you may never be able to win the battle of the bulge.

The six drugs that are forcing you to pack on the pounds are:

#1: Antidepressants

Antidepressant medications are notorious for causing people to put on weight. Medical experts found that up to 25 percent of patients who took these medications experienced weight gain.

Several different categories of these medications are associated with weight gain, including SSRI drugs (like Paxil and Prozac), MAO inhibitors (like Azilect and Marplan), and tricyclic antidepressants (like Doxepin and Norpramin).

Researchers have been arguing for years about why antidepressants trigger weight gain. They certainly can make you lethargic or fatigued, which won't do wonders for your exercise routine. They also may be affecting your metabolism at a cellular level.

If you experience a troubling weight gain while taking antidepressant drugs, talk to your doctor to discuss a change of medication to one with less risk.

#2: Beta blockers

Beta blockers are used to treat high blood pressure and certain types of heart problems. Some, but not all, beta-blocking medications can cause increased weight gain and difficulty losing weight. Atenolol and metoprolol are especially notorious for being linked to weight gain.

#3: Birth control pills or hormone replacement therapy

If you're a bit older, there's a good chance that birth control pills have been out of your life for some time—but you may be getting hormone replacement.

Changes in hormone levels can often result in weight gain. If you experience difficulty losing weight while taking these medications, talk to your doctor about changing doses or even trying different hormone brands.

Many alternative doctors recommend bioidentical hormone replacement therapy (instead of synthetic) because they believe it's safer and more closely mimics that natural hormones your body produces.

#4: Corticosteroids

Corticosteroid drugs include such medications as cortisone, hydrocortisone and Prednisone. They are used to treat a variety of medical conditions that involve inflammation and swelling, such as arthritis, asthma, allergies, lupus, and severe skin reactions.

They work by imitating the effects of adrenal hormones and are often prescribed to suppress immune system response. However, these drugs often have a number of side effects that make long-term use unworkable. Weight gain is one of these common effects.

Especially if you have joint problems, there are plenty of natural inflammation-fighters that are worth trying instead, like curcumin.

#5: Anti-psychotic medications

Individuals with schizophrenia and related conditions may find that their anti-psychotic medication causes them to put on weight.

Unfortunately, almost all anti-psychotic drugs cause this problem. If a change of medication is not able to manage the problem, your doctor may recommend a special weight loss program. High-protein, low-carb diets are often recommended for a variety of people suffering from mental and emotional issues.

#6: Anti-seizure drugs

If you have epilepsy or other condition that causes seizures, your anti-convulsive medication may be causing you to keep on excess weight. Drugs such as Depakote and Tegretol are known to have this effect.

A change of medication is often necessary to help you lose the extra weight caused by your drugs.

Lose Weight *4 Different Ways* with This Cooking Oil Trick

If your weight has been going up and down more than the stock market, you've probably had the same wish as many of your fellow dieters.

Wouldn't it be great if losing weight was just a little easier? What if you could just click your heels like Dorothy in the "Wizard of Oz" and watch the fat melt away?

Well, shedding pounds isn't that easy—but we may have the next best thing. Because it turns out the making one simple change to how you cook could help you drop weight fast.

In fact, just substituting coconut oil into your cooking routine could help you lose stubborn fat in at least four different ways. Coconut oil has now been scientifically proven to:

#1: Super-charge your metabolism

Coconut oil contains medium-chained fatty acids (MCFAs). Research published by the *American Journal of Clinical Nutrition* shows that these fatty acids can increase the metabolic rate by up to 48 percent in healthy-weight and overweight people, and up to 65 percent for obese people.

Although the effect only lasts about 24 hours, it can be helpful if your metabolism has been damaged by prolonged dieting or stress. Plus, if you're using coconut oil every day, you may get a continuous effect.

#2: Give your energy levels a boost

The MCFAs in coconut oil are easier for your liver to metabolize and convert to energy than the long-chain fatty acids in other oils. This means that less of the oil is stored as fat and more of it is used to supply energy for all your body's systems.

Taking 2 to 3 tablespoons of coconut oil every day can provide fuel to fight fatigue and keep you energized all day. You'll also be more likely to exercise when you're not feeling tired and worn out.

#3: Keep your hunger and cravings under control

Hunger is the body's signal that it needs more fuel, but eating more calories than you need leads to weight gain. The medium-chain triglycerides (MCTs) in coconut oil can help prevent overeating by keeping hunger in check.

When your body metabolizes MCTs, it produces ketone bodies which, according to several studies, have an appetite-reducing effect, especially when MCTs are eaten early in the day.

#4: Burn calories faster

To lose weight, you have to burn more calories than you take in. A study by the National Center for Biotechnology Information confirms that taking 15 to 30 grams (approximately 2 to 3 tablespoons) of coconut oil can help you burn an additional 120 calories per day.

Simply replacing your cooking fat with coconut oil can

help you burn more calories and help you achieve a deficit. However, any more than 2 to 3 tablespoons will simply add to your caloric intake and won't increase the calorie-burning effect.

Coconut oil is available at more supermarkets these days. If you want to buy it online, check out Spectrum Naturals Coconut Oil at **www.iherb.com**.

Use This Weird Shopping List to Melt Away Fat

When you're trying to lose weight, entering a supermarket is a little like walking into a war zone.

There are foods all around you loaded with sugars, additives, and other unhealthy chemicals that are just waiting to add inches to your waist.

But it doesn't have to be that way. In fact, there are simple and delicious foods that are proven to help you melt away fat. Here are some you need to add to your shopping list right away:

Fat-Fighter #1: Eggplants

While vegetables are important to any diet, you are better off eating non-starchy varieties if you want to lose weight. Non-starchy vegetables are full of fiber, so they help to satisfy your hunger.

Vegetables in this category include eggplant, onions, mushrooms, sweet peppers, and hot peppers.

Fat-Fighter #2: Spinach

Spinach was good enough for Popeye, and it's good enough for you, too. Eating leafy vegetables can help to reduce your daily intake of calories by helping you feel fuller. Leafy greens that make it to the list of foods you should eat include spinach, kale, mustard greens, collard greens, and lettuce.

Fat-Fighter #3: Broccoli

Packed full of nutrients, cruciferous vegetables are low in calories and high in flavor. This grouping of vegetables includes broccoli, Brussel sprouts, cauliflower, and cabbage.

Plus, studies have found that broccoli in particular is loaded with compounds that can help prevent heart disease.

Fat-Fighter #4: Raspberries

Eating raw fruits can help you to feel less hungry because they are full of fiber (plus lots of healthy antioxidants).

Believe it or not, the fruit with the most fiber is raspberries, with 8 grams per cup. Apples, bananas, oranges, and strawberries are other high-fiber fruits, with around 3–4 grams per serving.

Fat-Fighter #5: Almonds

You've probably heard that nuts like almonds are great for your heart—but they're important for your weight-loss efforts, too. Because nuts are full of protein and they take longer to digest, they help you feel full.

There's even some evidence that nuts help you burn more calories when you're just sitting around, doing nothing.

Ideally, you should select nuts in their raw form, and avoid nuts that have been roasted in oil.

Fat-Fighter #6: Beans

Legumes like beans are filled with hunger-busting fiber, and they're low in calories. This category includes peas, beans, lentils, peanuts, soybeans, and carobs. Legumes are often eaten as a single vegetable, but you can also include them in soups, stews, and salads.

Too Tired to Exercise? Try This Bodybuilder's Trick

When you're trying to lose weight and get in shape, sometimes the biggest challenge is getting off the couch.

You feel so drained of energy that the idea of going to the gym—or even taking the dog for a walk around the block—is the last thing on your mind.

But there's a simple supplement that can give you all the energy you need and could even make your workouts more effective.

And we may have the bodybuilding community to thank for it.

It's called L-carnitine, and it's an amino acid that is synthesized in the liver and kidneys. When you're young, your body makes all the L-carnitine it needs—but we tend to get deficient as we age.

And when you're deficient, you'll start noticing symptoms like lethargy, increased body fat, muscle loss, and even mental fog.

In other words, lots of symptoms that keep you from looking and feeling your best.

Bodybuilders have been taking L-carnitine supplements for years to build muscle and to get the energy they need for their marathon workouts. But supplementing with L-carnitine has plenty of benefits for seniors, too.

Here are just some of the benefits that you can get from taking L-carnitine.

#1: Increased energy

Your mitochondria are your cells' natural energy factories. And reduced mitochondrial function is one of the reasons people have less energy as they grow older.

L-carnitine is necessary for the transportation of fatty acids into your cells' mitochondria, where they are converted to energy. In other words, supplementing with carnitine can provide your body with what it needs to produce more energy.

#2: Reduced fat

The fact that you have more energy from supplementing with L-carnitine will help you to exercise more (one of the reasons bodybuilders take it). The extra work done by your muscles translates to more fat being burned. Many scientists believe that L-carnitine's role in transporting fat to cells also increases the rate at which fat is burned.

#3: Better heart function

Even mainstream heart doctors are (slowly) seeing the light on L-carnitine, especially when it comes to people with angina.

Angina is when you get discomfort or pain in the chest because your heart is unable to get enough oxygenated blood. You can use carnitine alongside conventional angina treatments to treat the condition more effectively.

It can help to reduce symptoms so that a person with angina

can exercise without chest pain. L-carnitine supplementation also may reduce symptoms of heart failure.

#4: Increased muscle mass

Most of us will start to lose muscle mass once we hit our thirties. The age-related loss of muscle is called "sarcopenia with aging." Sarcopenia with aging is especially problematic for people who live sedentary lives.

You can help to combat this problem by supplementing with L-carnitine. L-carnitine can improve your capacity for exercise while making it feel less difficult. The higher levels of L-carnitine decrease pain and limit lactic acid production.

#5: Shorter recovery time

L-carnitine can shorten the time it takes to recover from exercise. The buildup of lactic acid is one of the factors in recovery time and can cause muscle pain. L-carnitine can help you to produce less lactic acid and help you to get it out of your body in less time.

You can pick up 500 mg. L-carnitine supplements from Optimum Nutrition at **www.optimumnutrition.com**

This "Tea in a Pill" is a Weight-Loss Breakthrough

We've all heard about the health marvels of green tea. It's a bona fide super drink that can help improve everything from your heart to your brain.

But now studies are proving that green tea (and the compounds in it) may be the secret to turning your body into a fat-burning machine.

Of course, you have to make sure you're getting it the right way—and we'll explain exactly how in a moment.

But first let's take a second to understand the remarkable science behind this fat-melting breakthrough.

Most experts agree green tea's ability to promote weight loss comes from a specific type of antioxidant called catechins, especially epigallocatechin gallate (EGCG).

Studies show EGCG is responsible for relaying messages from the nervous system that encourage the body to start breaking down fat cells and using them as a source of energy.

The fat-burning abilities of green tea have been proven by numerous studies, one of which was conducted at the University of Medicine in Berlin, Germany.

Six overweight men took part in the two-day study. All of the subjects received two (300 mg) doses of EGCG, each dose separated by a 24-hour period.

After examining the data, the researchers concluded: "*These findings suggest that EGCG alone has the potential to increase fat oxidation in men and may thereby contribute to the anti-obesity effects of green tea.*"

A study conducted at the University of Birmingham in England also proved green tea's fat-burning abilities. The researchers recruited a group of young men, all of whom were in good health, and monitored their fat oxidation and tolerance to glucose during exercise.

The results showed the men who were given green tea burned an impressive **17 *percent more*** fat than the placebo group.

A longer study, conducted at Khon Kaen University in Thailand, produced equally impressive results. The study lasted for three months and 60 obese people took part.

At the end of the study, the subjects who'd been supplementing with green tea had burned 183 calories more per day than the placebo group.

Green tea can help you burn more calories and jumpstart your weight-loss efforts, and you should add it to your daily routine.

Of course, getting enough green tea to reap all the benefits can be a challenge. And that's where supplements come in.

You can get a concentrated dose of green tea and its healthy EGCG by taking green tea supplements.

Nature's Bounty makes a 315 mg. green tea supplement (similar to doses used in studies) that you can pick up at **www.pharmapacks.com.**

CHAPTER 13:

HAVE SEX LIKE A TEENAGER AGAIN WITH THESE SECRET LIBIDO BOOSTERS

The "Man Root" Secret to Mind-Blowing Sex After 60

Sex wasn't just great in your 20s.

It was easy, too, right?

It didn't matter if it was midnight or 3 p.m. on a Saturday—when you needed to perform, you were ready fast.

But it feels like once you reach a certain age, it can take a bit longer to be ready to perform—and sometimes you're not able to at all.

That can be embarrassing, frustrating, and put a real damper on your relationship.

But before you go running to your doctor for that "little blue pill," there's something out of Korea you might want to try first. In fact, it may even help you...

Roll back YEARS on your sexual odometer

Imagine being able to get—and keep—an erection whenever you want, for as long as you want. These are the kinds of results many guys have seen using Korean red ginseng.

Korean red ginseng (sometimes called Asian ginseng or

"Man root") is a powerful herbal remedy that's been used in traditional Asian healing for centuries to improve alertness and even as an aphrodisiac.

And if you're a guy looking to heat things up in the bedroom again, Korean red ginseng may be the answer to your prayers.

In a 2007 study out of Brazil's Sao Paulo University, 60 guys with erectile dysfunction took either 1,000 mg. of Korean red ginseng three times a day, or placebo, for 12 weeks.

And the difference was *amazing*!

Two-thirds of the guys taking Korean red ginseng reported significant improvements in the quality of their erections.

And these were improvements where it really counts, like firmness, penetration, and the ability to maintain their erections.

These guys must have felt 20 or 30 years younger in bed!

Imagine what these kinds of improvements could mean for YOU and your sex life.

And this wasn't a one-time thing, either. A major analysis out of Korea, published in 2008, looked at seven different studies on Korean red ginseng and erectile dysfunction, and found that it consistently improved symptoms.

Of course, with the erectile dysfunction drug market expected to hit $3 billion in the coming years, don't expect to hear about Korean red ginseng from the mainstream or drug companies anytime soon.

Now, of course, this leaves one BIG question -- what about the ladies? For ages, Big Pharma has been forgetting that there are millions of older women who could use a boost in the bedroom, too.

Well, it looks like Korean red ginseng can come to the rescue there, too.

In a study out of Korea's prestigious Chonnam National

University Medical School, 32 menopausal women took either 1 g. of Korean red ginseng a day or placebo. The women who took Korean red ginseng ended up experiencing improved sexual function with absolutely no side effects.

The authors concluded that Korean red ginseng had, "improved sexual arousal in menopausal women."

That's right—better, hotter sex without ANY side effects!

Aside from being rich in nutrients, Korean red ginseng is a natural adaptogen. That means it helps your body better cope with physical and emotional stress (which also can improve mental function).

And the inflammation and cortisol that your body produces during stress can be like poison for your sex life, whether you're a man or a woman.

If you've ever tried to perform sexually while you were really worried about something or stressed out, you know exactly what we're talking about. Stress can kill a love-making session before it even begins.

While most mainstream doctors never tell their patients about the power of Korean red ginseng, it's easy enough to take matters into your own hands.

You can buy Prince of Peace Korean Red Ginseng (without additives or fillers) at **www.puritan.com**.

Banish ED with These 5 PROVEN Remedies

Sex is an important part of any relationship. But when you can't perform, even the most intimate moments can turn embarrassing in a hurry.

The drug companies have made a fortune selling guys dangerous pills for erectile dysfunction like Viagra and Cialis. But these meds can come with serious side effects and some men can't take them at all.

But there are proven, natural supplements that can help get things working "down there" again. In fact, they're being used all over the world right now in countries where Big Pharma doesn't have a monopoly on the health care system.

Here are 5 natural ED remedies that can help restore your sex life—without risking your good health in the process:

ED Remedy #1: Horny goat weed

True to its name, horny goat weed is an herb that has been used for hundreds of years as an aphrodisiac.

According to Chinese legend, horny goat weed earned its name when a goat herder noticed that his goats started having more sex after consuming this herb.

Similar to Viagra, horny goat weed inhibits the PDE-5 enzyme. Inhibiting this enzyme causes the smooth muscles in the penis to relax while increasing blood flow. Another important component of this herb is icarin, which relaxes smooth muscle tissue.

You can buy horny goat weed from Piping Rock Health Products at **www.pipingrock.com**.

ED Remedy #2: Asian ginseng

Asian ginseng has been used for thousands of years to treat many health conditions, including ED. A double-blind placebo-controlled study performed by Brazilian researchers at the São Paulo University found that participants who ingested Asian ginseng demonstrated significant improvements in erectile function.

You can pick up Nature's Way Asian Ginseng at **www.iherb.com.**

ED Remedy #3: Maca root

Maca, another ancient herb, was used by the Incans to enhance stamina and energy. Maca root was also used by the ancient Peruvians to increase sex drive and cure infertility. For men who have lower than normal sperm counts, maca root amplifies the quantity of sperm.

A 2008 study from *CNS Neuroscience & Therapeutics* found that maca root helps treat erectile dysfunction caused by SSRIs (selective-serotonin reuptake inhibitors), which are commonly prescribed antidepressants.

Pick up maca root supplements at **www.pipingrock.com**.

ED Remedy #4: Ginkgo biloba

Because ginkgo biloba raises blood blow to the penis and relaxes the smooth muscles, it is another effective natural remedy for treating erectile dysfunction. Like maca root, ginkgo is very effective for people who are suffering from erectile dysfunction as a side effect of antidepressants.

In fact, in a study out of the University of California, San Francisco, ginkgo biloba improved sexual dysfunction in an impressive 76 percent of guys.

You can buy ginkgo supplements at **www.nowfoods.com.**

ED Remedy #5: Fo-ti root

Fo-ti root, native to China, has been used traditionally to prolong or restore youthful appearance and vitality. Is it any surprise that fo-ti root is a great treatment for erectile dysfunction? This herb acts as an aphrodisiac by preventing premature ejaculation, boosting blood supply to the penis, and dilating the capillaries.

Go to **www.naturesanswer.com** to see where you can buy the company's liquid Fo-ti supplement near you.

The "Under the Sea" Fix for Vaginal Dryness

When it comes to sexual performance, the problems aren't just limited to men.

Especially once they hit menopause and estrogen levels plummet, many women start experiencing severe vaginal dryness. That can make sex uncomfortable or even downright painful.

Lots of women turn to estrogen therapy or even messy lubes to try to fix the problem. But if you're dealing with dryness, there's a simple (and delicious) option you may want to try first.

The easy fix is oysters, and you probably know that they've been considered a natural aphrodisiac for hundreds of years. But they also may be the next promising solution for vaginal dryness.

You see, oysters are full of D-aspartic acid and NMDA, two compounds that can help trigger the release of sex hormones. And that produces a result you can notice—especially "down-stairs" where it counts.

Better still, oysters are a great natural source of zinc, which is an important component of vaginal lubricant. Studies have shown that zinc deficiency can block fatty acid pathways in your body, which can keep skin and tissues (including vaginal tissue) dry and uncomfortable.

In fact, a clinical review published in the prestigious medical journal *BMJ* found that nutritional deficiencies, like being low in zinc, may be the greatest contributor to sex problems for women.

Plus, women with higher levels of zinc have been shown to have higher sex drives, so oysters can give your libido a natural boost.

Now, of course, the biggest issue with oysters is their price. But if you want to give zinc a try, you can also get a good supply from red meat or even simple (and affordable) pumpkin seeds. Plus, there are plenty of zinc supplements available on the market.

And if you want to add some more fuel to the fire, try incorporating vitamin E into your supplement regimen. Vitamin E is especially effective because it works to help hydrate your vagina's mucous membranes.

Finally, it's important to avoid common causes of vaginal dryness that can make the problem worse. Douches and bubble baths can both contribute to dryness, so try laying off of them for a while as you give oysters or supplements a chance to work.

Is This Popular Med DESTROYING Your Manhood?!?

If you're struggling with erectile dysfunction, you've probably tried just about everything to fix the problem.

It seems like there's someone waiting around every corner to sell you some pump or gadget, or even that "little blue pill."

But it turns out that the REAL cause of your ED may be a lot simpler than you ever imagined.

In what's turning out to be a nightmare for the drug companies, studies are now proving that blood pressure drugs...medications that have made Big Pharma a fortune...are leaving guys with embarrassing cases of ED.

And lots of men never realize how potentially dangerous these meds are until it's too late.

One study involved more than 100 men who were being treated for hypertension at a clinic.

And a **whopping *68 percent*** said they were suffering from some form of ED—and nearly half of those cases were severe.

Can you imagine that? A nearly 70 percent chance of some form of ED once you start popping these pills.

Bet you never heard about that in your doctor's office or in those drug commercials, right?

The biggest problems seemed to come from diuretics and beta blockers, which are two of the most commonly prescribed classes of drugs for high blood pressure.

In fact, another study published out of Egypt in 2015 found that the beta blocker atenolol (sold under the brand name Tenormin) decreased the blood flow to penises of guys who were being treated.

These were men who didn't smoke, weren't diabetic, and were perfectly healthy—except that they had high blood pressure and were being treated for it.

And a German study found that metoprolol, sold under the brand names Lopressor and Toprol, caused erection problems in as little as 8 weeks.

Imagine the damage these drugs can do once you've been taking them for years!

Even many doctors are starting to agree that high blood pressure is one of the most overtreated conditions around. They can't even agree on what the definition of high blood pressure is!

If you're taking blood pressure meds and are suffering from ED, make a doctor's appointment right away. Talk about alternatives that may not cause such serious sexual side effects.

Or better still, flip to the heart section of this book for ways to lower your blood pressure naturally—no drugs required.

Get "In the Mood" (and *Stay* In the Mood) with the Cincinnati Secret

We've all been there. You're cozying up with your spouse in the bedroom at night, and the conditions are perfect for love-making.

But as you roll over for a little bit of foreplay, you hear those dreaded words.

"I'm not in the mood."

Loss of sexual desire is a major problem in relationships, especially as we get older. But a landmark study out of Cincinnati has now proven that a simple, ancient remedy may be the secret to getting your libido back.

And the best part? You can feel the difference in just weeks.

In a study led by Good Samaritan Hospital in Cincinnati, a small group of middle-aged women suffering from hypoactive sexual desire disorder (low sex drive) agreed to try acupuncture for 5 weeks.

Acupuncture is a Chinese remedy that's been used for thousands of years to treat a variety of health conditions, including sexual problems. It's been shown to stimulate the body's healing response and increase blood flow throughout the body.

And despite what you may have heard, it's a relatively painless procedure that many people come to love and enjoy.

And after just 5 weeks of twice-weekly treatment, the women in the study reported "significant increases in sexual function, especially desire."

They even reported better orgasms!

That sounds pretty good, right? Now just imagine if the study had gone on even longer!

And, believe it or not, acupuncture can have lots of sexual benefits for men, too.

In a four-week Dutch study published in the *International Journal of Impotence Research*, acupuncture helped some men have more sex and improve the quality of their erections.

In fact, nearly a third of men reported they were getting frisky more often with their partners.

The acupuncture sessions only lasted 30 minutes (who doesn't have half an hour to improve their sex life?) and the needles were only applied to eight different stimulating points throughout the body.

Talk about simple, fast, and effective!

Finally, a 2013 study from Canada found that acupuncture could help restore sex drive in people taking prescription antidepressants. And we all know that these drugs can wipe out your libido fast.

If you're looking to jumpstart your sex life and give acupuncture a try, look for a medical acupuncturist. The American Academy of Medical Acupuncture can help you find a practitioner near you.

Just check out their website at **www.medicalacupuncture.org.** And remember—acupuncture may be covered by your insurance plan.

These 3 Superfoods Are Like *Jumper* Cables for Your Sex Drive

Sex after 60 can be the greatest sex of your life—your body just needs a little more preparation first.

And getting your body ready for sex starts with eating the right foods. We're not talking about loading up on tofu or eating like a health nut, either.

There are three easy and simple foods you can start incorporating into your diet today that can help give your body the fuel it needs for the kind of toe-curling sex both you and your partner deserve.

Sex Fuel #1: Flaxseed

You can buy flaxseed just about anywhere, and it's easy to sprinkle on a salad or even incorporate into baking. And it's absolutely LOADED with zinc and omega-3 fatty acids.

Zinc is renowned for increasing testosterone and sperm count, and omega-3 improves sexual function by increasing the amount of blood that flows to the sexual organs.

To further increase your intake of omega-3 fatty acids, look into fatty fish like sardines and salmon. You can also enjoy nuts like almonds that are great sources of omega-3s.

Sex Fuel #2: Pomegranate juice

Like flaxseed, pomegranate juice can also lower the risk of erectile dysfunction. And if you have children or grandchildren who are trying to conceive, pomegranate juice can increase the quality of sperm and a man's sperm count.

Sex Fuel #3: Garlic

Garlic is not only known for being one of the top fertility foods for men, it is also a sexual super food.

Garlic contains allicin, which is great for increasing the amount of blood that flows to the penis. Another compound in garlic, S-allyl cysteine was shown in a study out of China to reverse erectile dysfunction in diabetic rats.

And if you have diabetes, you know it's a major risk factor for ED.

The best part about garlic is its taste—and it's easy to add to lots of different foods. But of you're not a fan of garlic, supplements are widely available and dirt cheap.

You can pick up concentrated garlic supplements at **www.vitacost.com** for well less than $10 a month.

This isn't some crazy or restrictive diet we're recommending here. These are 3 foods that are easy to add to just about any eating plan.

On your next trip to the supermarket, pick up some fresh flaxseed, pomegranate juice and garlic, and work them into your meals. They should produce a difference you'll feel in the bedroom—and that your spouse will LOVE.

Send Your Sex Life SOARING With This Sacred Mountain Root

This Libido-Booster Works Fast for Both Men AND Women.

How about a second honeymoon?

I'm not talking about cashing in your airline miles... emptying your bank account...or taking a trip to the beach.

I'm talking about the romance.

Remember those passionate nights of sheet-twisting love-making that left you both satisfied—*and hungry for more?*

You can have nights like that again...in facts, lots of seniors already are. Because they've discovered...

The underground secret to the best sex of your life—in just two weeks FLAT!

No more little blue pills. No more embarrassing performance problems. And no more feeling like you're just "not in the mood."

This sexual breakthrough works for both men AND women—and it may hold the key to unlocking sexual drive and performance like you haven't seen in years.

The "Mountain Secret" to GREAT Sex

This sex-boosting discovery is called **maca root**—and don't go looking for it in your backyard.

It grows in some of the highest and most inhospitable parts of the Andes Mountains in South America. And while maca root is a chore to harvest, its effects are absolutely mind-blowing.

The Incas started using maca root as a source of energy and strength more than 3,000 years ago.

And while that boost of energy and strength helped the Incas survive long treks and hunting expeditions, it also comes in mighty handy in the bedroom.

But unlike nearly all of the sex drugs on the market today, maca root delivers a major libido boost for *both* sexes. That means you and your spouse can jumpstart your sex drives together!

So how powerful is this Peruvian plant?

In a study published in the *CHS Neuroscience & Therapeutics* journal, researchers tested maca root on men and women whose sex drives had been destroyed by antidepressants.

"Maca root will make you feel like you're in the prime of your life! And it's not just for men, either."

And if you take these drugs, you know that's a MAJOR side effect.

But after just two weeks of taking 3 mg. of maca root a day, both men and women saw HUGE improvements in their sex drives.

What would that mean for you, your spouse, and your relationship?

Another study even tested maca root on 57 men with performance problems, like erectile dysfunction.

And the results were practically IDENTICAL. The men taking 3 mg. a day saw ***big increases in their sexual desire and*** *performance in just weeks.*

Who says you can't feel young again—at least in the bedroom?

The "Passion Smoothie" You Can Share With Your Spouse

Maca root is most potent in its powdered form. That's when it contains the most nutrients—and you can measure exactly how much you're getting.

And it's incredibly easy to mix into a delicious smoothie. That means you can start each day getting your body ready for a night of passion.

This Blueberry Maca Smoothie is great for men and women. And, in addition to maca, you'll get a strong dose of antioxidants and vitamins that are critical for a healthy sex life.

Ingredients:

- 3 mg—Maca Root Powder
- ½ cup—Blueberries
- 1-2—Bananas
- 1 cup—Almond Milk
- 1 tspn—Cinnamon
- 1-2 tspn—Vanilla Extract
- ½ cup—Vanilla Yogurt

Instructions:

- Combine almond milk, yogurt, and maca root powder in blender.
- Blend briefly.
- Add blueberries, bananas, and cinnamon.
- Blend until smooth.
- If needed, add more almond milk or water to achieve desired consistency.

- Sprinkle in cinnamon and vanilla extract and blend again.
- Sample smoothie and add more cinnamon and vanilla extract to taste.
- Enjoy the perks of a nutritional and libido-enhancing beverage!

Four Powerful Sex-Boosters

So, how does maca root work its magic? Well, it's jam-packed with nutrients and compounds that boost your sex drive and performance in at least four different ways.

Sex Booster #1: Maca root contains plant sterols which increase testosterone in both men and women. And that jump-starts passion and desire for both sexes.

Now we tend to think of testosterone as a male hormone, but it's vital for women's libido, too.

But, ladies, don't worry. Research has shown that maca root (even taken over a long period of time) won't change your hormone profile in any permanent way

Sex Booster #2: Maca root has a compound called p-methoxybenzyl isothiocyanate that appears to be exclusive to plant. It naturally enhances libido, and studies show it even protect you from cancer.

Sex Booster #3: This powerful plant has high levels glucosinolates, which are important for controlling mation and detoxifying our bodies (which are both for sexual health). Glucosinolates also seem to protect certain sexual organ diseases, like cancer.

Sex Booster #4: Maca root is also loaded with amino acids, vitamin C, iron, potassium, copper mins, which are all critical to feeling healthy, "in the mood."

If you're suffering from an absent sex drive, you have nothing to lose. Maca root could have your passion restored in as little as two weeks with just 3 mg a day.

Its mild, earthy taste makes it easy to incorporate into your daily routine.

Maca root powder pairs well with chocolate or vanilla and disappears into coffee, tea, smoothies, and shakes.

And now that maca root is becoming more well known, it can be found at health food stores among other vitamins and supplements.

But it is crucial to find a pure source because even the highest quality maca root can contain a type of mold that grows during the drying process.

When you buy maca, get it from a high-end brand—even if it costs a bit more. Pure maca will leave you energized and

Some of the best brands are: **The Maca Team** which sells powdered, liquid, and capsulated maca, and **Z Natural Foods'** raw organic powder. You can find both of these brands easily online.

Can American "Liberty Weed" Jumpstart Your Sex Drive Again?

He was one of America's most important founding fathers—you'll even see his face adorning our $100 bill.

But there's one place you're never going to see Ben Franklin's smiling mug or portly profile—and that's on the cover of *Men's Health* magazine.

Franklin was balding, overweight, and 70 years old when the Declaration of Independence was signed. But Franklin had a secret that left many of his peers absolutely speechless…

He was a total sex machine, able to satisfy women decades younger!

Franklin was reported to have bedded countless women during his senior years. And his flirtations may have even played a role in helping to secure French support during the Revolutionary War.

Time magazine even called him a "babe magnet."

So what was Franklin's secret? And how can you put it to work to enjoy the best sex of your life during your senior years?

Well, Franklin (and some other sexed-up founding fathers)

may have been getting a little help.

And it came from a powerful herbal remedy known as American ginseng—or what we call "Liberty Weed."

American ginseng is a proven libido-booster—and it looks like Franklin was no stranger to its powers.

Franklin is actually credited with introducing the American colonists to ginseng, and encouraging its cultivation. He described the plant as having "wonderful" virtues, and even Thomas Jefferson grew it on his estate.

And when it comes to giving a boost to your sexual performance, science proves that the virtues of American ginseng are wonderful, indeed.

A massive analysis published by Hong Kong researchers in 2013 found that in animal studies, ginseng was found to increase sexual activity, boost testosterone, and even increase the quality of sperm.

Talk about a triple threat!

And the powers of ginseng don't end there.

Randomized clinical trials—a gold standard in medical research—found that American ginseng and its cousin, Korean ginseng, were effective at improving erectile dysfunction.

A study from the University of Naples in Italy concluded that ginseng, "enhances physical performance (including sexual), promotes vitality and increases resistance to stress and aging."

Ginseng is a powerful antioxidant and is effective at controlling inflammation—and inflammation can kill both sex drive and performance fast.

Ginseng is a time-tested herbal remedy that's been used safely for hundreds of years. If you're looking to give yourself a boost in the bedroom, it's a solution worth trying.

You can pick up Swanson Premium American Ginseng in 550 mg capsules at **www.swansonvitamins.com**.

CHAPTER 14:

THE NATURAL HEALERS' GUIDE TO GETTING "BRICK HARD" BONES

Don't TOUCH Another Calcium Tablet (Until You Do This First)!

It's the sham mainstream advice that older women have been getting for decades—a calcium pill a day keeps bone loss away.

We've all been told how important calcium is for our bones, and how it's an important building block for bone tissue.

But there's a lot more to the story as far as calcium is concerned—and taking straight calcium could have serious long-term effects for both your brain and your heart.

That doesn't mean you need to completely stop taking calcium—you just need to change how you're taking it.

First, the bad news.

A recent study shows that women who suffer from cerebrovascular disease are up to **seven times more likely** to suffer from dementia when taking a calcium supplement.

Cerebrovascular disease occurs when blood vessels in the brain become blocked by fat or cholesterol (it can often be triggered by atherosclerosis). This loss of blood flow can damage the brain and lead to dangerous conditions like dementia or stroke.

For the study, researchers followed a group of dementia-free women ages 70–92 for a five-year period. Over the course of the study, the researchers monitored their use of calcium supplements and tracked whether they were diagnosed with dementia.

That's how scientists found dementia risk increased by about sevenfold in women with cerebrovascular disease when taking calcium supplements.

Now, that may be a lot different from everything you've heard about calcium before. Millions of women just like you are taking calcium every day to protect their bones.

But the fact is, when calcium enters your body, it can go to either your bones or your arteries, where it can lead to plaque buildup.

Calcium needs helpers to get to your bones and not your arteries—specifically, vitamins D3 and K2.

That's something you *never* hear in all those ads for calcium supplements. But vitamin K2 helps direct calcium into your bones and away from your arteries, and vitamin D3 helps your bones absorb it.

That means that taking calcium on its own may not help your bone health as much as you think—and, according to this latest research, can come with significant risks.

But taking this powerful nutrient combo of D3 and K2 (you can buy these vitamins through most online vitamin retailers or at your local health store) along with calcium can help direct the calcium where it belongs—to your bones.

Hushed-Up NASA Discovery Stops Bone Loss

It's one of the greatest bone-health threats being faced by countless seniors today…and it's one that many of them have never been warned about.

It's not old age or some calcium deficiency—it's the radiation now being used in dozens of mainstream tests and treatments.

Whether you've been treated for cancer—or just have spent years getting X-rays, CT scans and mammograms—all that radiation can take a long-term toll on your bones, leaving them weak and brittle.

But in 2016, NASA discovered a simple breakthrough that can help keep your bones strong, even if you've been exposed to a whopping amount of radiation.

And believe it or not, it was barely covered by the mainstream media.

So what's this bone-health breakthrough? It's a special groups of compounds found in a fruit your mother always told you to eat more of.

Prunes.

You see, when astronauts are launched into space, they're exposed to enormous amounts of radiation. And space scientists have known for years that all this radiation can damage astronauts' bones.

Of course, your local radiologist knows this, too—but when was the last time you got a warning? Never?

Well, after exposing rats to simulated space radiation, the researchers investigated several treatments with anti-inflammatory or antioxidant properties that they thought could prevent the oxidative stress and bone damage that can lead to cancellous bone loss—or what's commonly called "spongy bone."

That's when your bones get porous and you're a sitting duck for a potentially serious fracture.

The treatments included dihydrolipoic acid, ibuprofen, an antioxidant cocktail and dried plums (prunes).

And it turned out that prunes had the power to stop bone loss, even after massive radiation doses.

Nancy Turner, one of the researchers involved, said that prunes are loaded with antioxidants and anti-inflammatories that can help avoid "loss of structural integrity" our bones face from radiation.

"From this study, we can conclude that inclusion of dried plums in the diet may prevent the skeletal effects of radiation exposures either in space or here on Earth," she wrote.

While this study focused on the extraterrestrial powers of prunes, there are other studies showing that these tiny fruits are also good for the bones of Earth-bound and radiation-free folks as well.

In fact, a study from San Diego State University showed that eating just five to six prunes a day could prevent and reverse bone loss in animals and humans alike.

Of course, when buying prunes, be sure to pick organic

varieties. Non-organic fruits and vegetables are regularly treated with pesticides that studies show can be harmful to your bones.

So if you're out shopping this weekend, do your bones a favor and pick up some prunes!

The Billion-Dollar Bone Drug You Should Throw in the Trash

If you're suffering from osteoporosis—or are at risk for it—you may have been sold a load of bull by the drug companies and the mainstream.

For years they've been promising they can solve your bone problems with a simple bone-building drug called Fosamax.

In fact, doctors are handing it out like Halloween candy to seniors—and you've probably seen commercials for it on TV.

But Fosamax comes with a dark secret that many doctors and drug executives would prefer you never learned about. In fact, studies show it could be setting you up for some of the worst bone problems of your life.

You see, researchers started noticing a rise in fractures of the femur (thighbone)—which is the longest, largest and strongest bone in our body.

It's a bone that should be hard to break—but if you're taking Fosamax, all bets may be off.

A study in the 2008 *Journal of Orthopedic Trauma* revealed a link between Fosamax and a rare type of fracture called an atypical subtrochanteric femur fracture, or a fracture that occurs just below the hip joint.

Of the 25 patients taking the drug, *two-thirds* of them suffered similar femoral fractures.

Those aren't odds that any senior—should accept.

And here's the worst part. The bones that broke didn't look like typical osteoporosis bones. In fact, they looked strong and healthy—but the bones broke anyway.

Of course, Big Pharma tried to fight these findings. But eventually the risk of femoral fractures was added to the list of Fosamax's possible side effects.

The Food and Drug Administration even published a Drug Safety Announcement in March of 2010 telling patients taking bisphosphonates drugs like Fosamax to talk to their doctors if they experience hip or thigh pain.

But it looks like the problems with Fosamax still aren't over.

In a study from the University of Southern California, researchers found that 4 percent of participants taking Fosamax suffered from a condition called osteonecrosis of the jaw, also known as "jawbone death."

"Here at the USC School of Dentistry, we're getting two or three new patients a week that have bisphosphonate-related osteonecrosis of the jaw—and I know we're not the only ones seeing it," Dr. Parish P. Sedghizadeh said.

But despite the problems with Fosamax, doctors keep prescribing it—even for people who don't have osteoporosis yet.

But research is proving that if you want to protect your bones—and your good health—Fosamax is one drug you need to get out of your medicine cabinet right away.

The 10-Cent Secret to Bones of Steel

When it comes to keeping bones strong—and preventing breaks that could rob you of your independence and quality of life—the mainstream medical establishment is like a one-trick pony.

All we ever hear about it's calcium, calcium, and more calcium.

But there's actually one super-mineral that may be even more important to your bones than calcium. It's available for pennies a day, and it could hold the secret to keeping bones steel-girder strong as you age.

This miracle mineral is magnesium, and it may be the greatest bone booster that many seniors still don't know about.

You may have heard about how great magnesium is for your heart…or even that it's called the "calming mineral" for helping to melt away stress.

But that may be nothing compared to what it does for your bones. In fact, about 60 percent of the magnesium in our bodies is stored in our bones!

Magnesium is like a general that helps direct bone-building nutrients and enzymes. It converts vitamin D to its active state so it can go to work building and supporting your bones.

Plus, it activates a key enzyme called calcitonin that helps to preserve your bone structure and prevent bone loss.

And the research behind magnesium deficiency and bone loss is staggering.

Studies have shown that being low in magnesium actually interferes with the hardening of the tissue matrix as your body generates new bone. Being low in magnesium also promotes inflammation, which is a major risk factor for osteoporosis and bone loss.

Research out of Japan, published in the prestigious *Journal of the American College of Nutrition* found that women with poor bone density were also significantly more likely to have the lowest levels of magnesium in their blood.

And the famous, multi-year Framingham Osteoporosis Study found that seniors who had the most magnesium in their diets suffered less bone loss over the four years measured.

Another study published in *Nutrition Reviews* found that women who were given magnesium supplements (as magnesium hydroxide) for two years had greater bone density and seemed to be at less risk for fractures.

And unlike lots of the other bone-builders on the market, magnesium supplements are unbelievably affordable.

You can buy Nature Made High-Potency Magnesium (400 mg.) for about $10 (or roughly 30 cents a day) from **www.luckyvitamin.com.**

If you want to add more magnesium to your diet, you can also load up on magnesium-rich foods like almonds, spinach, cashews, peanuts and black beans.

Skipping This Popular Bone Test Could Save Your Health

It arrives in the mail every year—that reminder from your doctor's office that it's time for your DXA bone scan.

For years we've been told that the DXA is the best way to catch osteoporosis early and to give us a fighting chance at saving our bones.

But there's a big secret with the DXA scan that many doctors' offices and imaging labs aren't as quick to advertise—and it's one that could jeopardize your health.

The fact is, the DXA may be the least reliable test in all of medicine today. And that's really saying something.

A growing army of researchers is even claiming that you're better off skipping the DXA completely.

One of the major problems with the DXA is that it doesn't take much to throw off the results. Things like clothing, fat, or even shadows on your bones can lead to inaccurate results and a diagnosis of a bone problem you don't have—and the machine has a margin of error of 5–6 percent to begin with.

And changes in bone mineral density happen very slowly

and are subject to a great deal of interpretation. That means you could get two completely different diagnoses from two different doctors.

And in lots of cases, the DXA can't reliably distinguish the changes in your bone density from one year to the next. In fact, one study found that getting a bone scan even once every 8 years didn't do a thing to improve patient outcomes.

And many doctors want you to get a DXA *every year*—and Medicare pays for it every two years.

The real danger is that an inaccurate DXA screening could lead you to be prescribed potentially dangerous bone-building bisphosphonate drugs like Fosamax that have been linked to side effects like heartburn, joint pain, dizziness, and even certain types of bone breaks!

As one study from the University of New Mexico reported, "Poor-quality BMD testing and reporting can result in inappropriate clinical decisions, causing unnecessary worry and expense for the patient and possible harm."

And as Dr. Catherine Burt Driver points out, there is very little evidence that the treatment changes made as a result of DXA scans will do anything to significantly reduce your risk of certain types of bone breaks.

So why does mainstream medicine keep pushing DXA scans? It's all about the money.

When doctors' offices or imaging centers buy equipment, they expect a return on their investment several times over. And at $200–$300 a pop, DXA scans are easy money.

But for the sake of your health—and your wallet—the DXA scan is one test you're better off skipping.

Don't Let This "Brain Pill" Eat Your Bones Away

They're mainstream medicine's version of "happy pills" being handed out to millions of patients as a magic cure for depression.

But the people who antidepressants are *really* making happy are the drug company executives who are making a fortune in profits.

You've probably heard plenty about the nasty side effects that come with antidepressants, like weight gain, loss of sex drive, and even suicidal thoughts.

But now multiple studies have shown that antidepressants could be Public Enemy #1 for your bones, and could put you on the fast track to a serious bone break.

One study out of Canada found that people taking selective serotonin reuptake inhibitors (SSRIs) like Lexapro, Paxil, Prozac and Zoloft DOUBLED their risk of suffering a fracture linked to bone loss.

SSRIs interfere with how the neurotransmitter serotonin moves throughout your body. But researchers believe that serotonin may play a big role in how healthy bone cells develop.

The research out of Canada should have sounded a major alarm as far as prescribing SSRIs to seniors is concerned.

But the bad news was just starting.

A study from the University of Minnesota, published in the *Archives of Internal Medicine*, looked at more than 2,700 senior women. It turns out that those taking SSRIs suffered from greater bone loss in their hips.

And if there's one place where you don't want to lose bone— or risk a fracture—it's in your hips.

A second study, published in the same issue of the *Archives of Internal Medicine*, produced eerily similar findings.

In that study, researchers analyzed health data for nearly 6,000 men aged 65 and older. And the men taking SSRIs had lower bone density in both their hips and in their lower spines.

Some researchers want the Food and Drug Administration to start requiring drug companies to study the effects of SSRIs on bone health before new medications are approved. But with all the influence that Big Pharma has over the FDA, there's little chance of that happening.

Your best bet is to look for ways to treat your depression naturally. Flip to the brain health chapter of this book for safe, natural treatments you can start using right away.

This Blacklisted Treatment Could Save Your Thinning Bones

If you've gone through menopause—or are going through it now—you know your estrogen levels can fall off a cliff.

That can produce some symptoms you're sure to notice right away, like hot flashes, mood swings, and even a loss of sex drive.

But that estrogen shortage can also create some serious health problems you won't notice right away, like thinning bones. Estrogen plays a critical role in accelerating the development of healthy new bone.

And a loss of estrogen is a major reason why so many older women end up with bone loss or even osteoporosis.

The easy answer is to replenish your estrogen levels through hormone replacement therapy (HRT). It can help protect your bones and many women treated with estrogen report that even their worst menopause symptoms vanish.

But if you've looked into estrogen replacement, you've probably learned the hard way that the mainstream medical establishment has been waging a decades-long war against HRT.

Their favorite line of attack is that certain cancers (like breast cancer) feed off of estrogen, and that estrogen therapy could make you a sitting duck for tumors.

But it looks like the science behind estrogen and cancer has a lot more to it than the mainstream would have you believe. In fact, as far as breast cancer is concerned, their arguments are paper-thin.

Research has shown that women taking HRT when they were diagnosed with breast cancer were actually more likely to survive their cancer.

And that's not all.

According to a study published in the *Journal of the National Cancer Institute*, estrogen therapy may even help women who've already been diagnosed with breast cancer.

In that study, women who received HRT after a breast cancer diagnosis—when many doctors are afraid to prescribe it—were half as likely to see their cancer come back, and two-thirds less likely to die from it!

Estrogen wasn't causing cancer in this study—it looks like it was preventing it.

And while many doctors are withholding HRT from women after a breast cancer diagnosis, Jack Cusick, PhD, a researcher from the Imperial Cancer Research Fund in London, says this study raises "doubts about the wisdom of this practice."

And research shows that skipping out on estrogen can be a real threat to your thinning bones.

A report from the Swiss Society Against Osteoporosis concluded that, "There is no doubting the efficacy of HRT for the primary prevention of osteoporosis in post-menopausal women."

And a two-year study on women found that even very low doses of estrogen resulted in significant increases in bone density.

When it comes to estrogen therapy, many alternative doctors recommend bioidentical hormones, which more closely resemble the hormones our bodies naturally produce.

To find a doctor who offers bioidentical HRT, a good place to start is the physician locator on the American College for Advancement in Medicine website (go to **www.acam.org** and look under the Resources tab).

If you want to try to boost estrogen levels on your own, try incorporating more soy into your diet. Soy contains chemicals called isoflavones that have a similar function and structure to estrogen.

A research analysis out of Japan found that menopausal women who took soy isoflavones saw significant increases in the bone mineral density in their lumbar spines.

There are plenty of soy-rich foods available, including kidney beans, lima beans, fava beans, and chickpeas. But you can also purchase soy isoflavones supplements.

You can pick up Nature's Way Soy Isoflavones at **www.iherb.com** or **www.jet.com**.

Weird Sea Creature Unlocks Secret to TOTAL ARTHRITIS RELIEF!

Slash Your Pain Levels 89% in Just 4 Weeks

If you're one of the 21 million Americans living with bad arthritis, you know it's not really "living" at all.

The pain in your fingers…or hips…or knees hits you first thing in the morning.

And it doesn't let up all day.

Complain to your doctor enough, and he may even prescribe you a powerful opioid painkiller like OxyContin or fentanyl… the same class of addictive drugs that are killing THOUSANDS of Americans a year.

Some choice, right? Either put up with your arthritis, or risk your life trying to mask the pain.

Well, believe it or not, on the other side of the world, they're not having this problem at all.

Because off the coast of New Zealand, scientists have discovered a breakthrough natural remedy that…

Reduces pain by 89 percent in just one month!

I'm talking about a bona fide CURE that's helping real people like you right now.

There's a good chance your doctor has never even heard of it…but getting your hands on this natural pain reliever is a lot easier than you'd think.

Miracle Pain Relief…in a Neon Shell?!

The green-lipped mussel is native only to the waters of New Zealand.

But its healing powers are making it famous all over the world.

Green-lipped mussels have a vivid green stripe along their outer edges…but that's not the only thing that makes them remarkable.

You've probably heard that omega-3 fatty acids, like the kind you find in fish oil, are crucial to pain relief and protecting your joint cells.

Well, green-lipped mussels contain more omega-3s than just about any food or product you'll find on the market.

In fact, lyprinol, a fatty acid compound found in green-lipped mussel extract is…

- 175 times more potent than Evening Primrose Oil
- 175 times more potent than Salmon Oil
- 200 times more potent than Flax Oil

Green-lipped mussel extract also contains seatone and furan fatty acids that have been proven to slash the out-of-control inflammation that is making so many arthritis sufferers' lives miserable.

And here's the best part…

This powerful undersea cure works **just like prescription pain-relief drugs**—but without all the risks and side effects!

That's because green-lipped mussel extract inhibits the COX and LOX enzyme pathways that cause inflammation throughout your body.

This is the EXACT SAME effect you'd get from prescription COX-2 inhibitors like Celebrex…but you don't have to worry about drug side effects like diarrhea, vomiting and high blood pressure.

Green-lipped mussel extract is simply one of the most powerful pain-fighters on the planet.

And it's one that could have you *nearly pain free in just one short month!*

89% Pain Relief? You'd Better Believe It!

A study from the Academic Clinical Hospital in Poland looked at the effects of green-lipped mussel extract and fish oil on folks like you suffering from arthritis.

And the results were amazing!

In fact, the patients taking mussel extract experienced an **89 percent decrease in pain and a 91 percent improvement in quality of life.**

And it took just four weeks!

What would it mean to you to be nearly pain-free in just one month? To be able to go for a walk…or play golf…or work in your garden without worrying about your arthritis leaving you in agony?

These are the types of results that real people…just like you…are experiencing right now with green-lipped mussel extract.

And this research out of Poland wasn't a one-hit wonder.

In 2003, an investigative study from Korea found that lyprinol alone improved joint function in **80 percent of arthritis** patients in eight weeks.

And in 2006, a *Clinical Rheumatology* journal review discovered that green-lipped mussel extract benefits both osteoarthritis and rheumatoid arthritis symptoms.

In fact, **75 percent of patients with both kinds of arthritis experienced reduced pain after just one month of mussel extract treatment.**

These are remarkable results! So why haven't you heard of them?

Prescription painkillers are a billion-dollar business in the United States. And the drug companies have no interest in promoting natural cures that won't give them a fortune in profits.

But green-lipped mussel extract…this powerful, natural pain reliever…is available to Americans like you RIGHT NOW.

If you know where to look.

Get Your Hands on this Undersea Miracle

If you or someone you love is suffering from the horrific symptoms of arthritis, give green-lipped mussel extract a try.

For rheumatoid arthritis, try 300–350 mg a day and 900–1,200 mg for osteoarthritis.

There is no precise recommended dosage, however, and up to 3,000 mg a day has been proven safe in studies.

For some, it will take mere days to feel a difference, and for others up to 8 weeks may be necessary. But stick with it…the results are worth it.

You can find green-lipped mussel extract in several forms.

There are capsules, available from **XtendLife** and **New Zealand Pure Health**. And there is mixable powder like the one from **NutriCargo**.

All have been proven effective against arthritis pain.

It Works For Your Pets, Too!

Green-lipped mussel extract has also been proven to safely improve arthritis pain in animals—from dogs and cats to livestock and horses!

In 2012, a team from New Zealand conducted a study on the effects of green-lipped mussel extract on horses with chronic osteoarthritis.

Over the course of 56 days, 19 horses were given the extract and 20 were given a placebo.

At the conclusion of the study, the horses given green-lipped mussel extract experienced a significant reduction in symptoms while the placebo group experienced none.

And 2013 Canadian study showed that mussel extract significantly improved motor activity and overall comfort for 30 dogs suffering from arthritis pain.

The research team even proposed that green-lipped mussels extract be recommended more frequently as a treatment for dogs with arthritis.

Manufacturers even make the extract specifically for our pets.

You can buy it in powder form from **Super Snouts** or as a treat from **The Honest Kitchen**.

CHAPTER 15:

10 HEALTH SECRETS YOU'LL *NEVER* SEE ON TV

Get "Eagle Eyes" With This Powerful Supplement Combo

Losing our eyesight is one of the most terrifying issues we face as we age.

It can start with something simple, like having trouble reading the fine print in the newspaper. And after a while, just driving a car or recognizing the faces of loved ones can become nearly impossible.

You don't deserve to spend your golden years slowly being robbed of your vision…and even your independence. And starting today, you may finally be able to put those worries behind you for good.

Because there are two powerful plant compounds that can help keep you safe from one of the most common causes of vision loss in seniors.

And you can start putting these powerful breakthroughs to work for you for just pennies a day!

Lutein and zeaxanthin are carotenoids, or powerful antioxidants that are found in foods like green, leafy vegetables and even eggs. And unlike a lot of other antioxidants, they actually go to work right in the retinas of your eyes.

In fact, research shows that…

Lutein and zeaxanthin can help stop vision loss… before it's too late

You see, age-related macular degeneration (AMD) occurs when you suffer damage to your macula, which is located in the center of your retina. That can nearly destroy your "central vision," or your ability to recognize things that are right in front of you.

AMD is a leading cause of vision loss among people over 50, according to the National Eye Institute. And losing your central vision can cost you your driver's license, make you more prone to tripping, slipping, or falling, and even make reading or recognizing faces a challenge.

But studies show that lutein and zeaxanthin hold the secret to preventing AMD and even slowing the progression of the disease.

In addition to delivering antioxidant power directly to your retinas, and protecting them from free radical damage, lutein and zeaxanthin also help shield your eyes from blue light damage.

We get exposed to blue light daily from our televisions, smartphones, computers, and even light bulbs, and over time this light can be damaging to our eyes.

But lutein and zeaxanthin nourish our eyes and provide powerful protection against this damage, and that can mean big results when it comes to AMD.

Research has shown that people who get enough lutein and zeaxanthin are less likely to develop AMD, which means they're critical to saving your vision.

In a study published in *Nutrition & Metabolism,* supplementing with lutein and zeaxanthin increased the density of macular pigment in the eyes of patients. And that's considered critical to preventing AMD from ever taking hold.

But if you already have AMD, lutein and zeaxanthin may be able to throw the brakes on the disease. In fact...

Lutein and zeaxanthin are so powerful, even our government was forced to admit they work!

In the Age-Related Eye Disease Study (AREDS2), sponsored by the federal National Eye Institute, researchers found that people who added lutein and zeaxanthin to their supplement regimen reduced the risk of their macular degeneration worsening by up to 25 percent!

That's up to a 25 percent greater chance of keeping your vision from deteriorating, without touching a prescription drug!

You can imagine these government researchers practically falling off their chairs!

And these are differences you're going to notice. In a study published in the journal *Optometry*, people who supplemented with 8 mg. of zeaxanthin daily for a year could drive better at night and see an average of 1.5 lines better on an eye chart!

They were actually *reversing* their AMD symptoms and improving their vision!

Now, getting more lutein and zeaxanthin from your diet is a great place to start.

Kale, spinach and collard greens are three of the best sources of lutein and zeaxanthin. But it can be tough to get enough from just diet alone—and odds are, you're not.

So if you're serious about protecting...and even saving... your eyesight, supplementing is critical. The good news is that there are supplements in the market that combine the powers of both lutein and zeaxanthin into one, easy-to-use formulation.

MacuGuard Ocular Support from Life Extension is one such supplement. It also offers the natural ingredient astaxanthin to help with eye fatigue.

You can get a 60-capsule bottle, enough for two months, at **www.lifeextension.com.**

You'll want to take lutein and zeaxanthin with fat to aid absorption.

Dirt-Cheap Supplement Fights Ugly Cold Sores

Is there anything more embarrassing?

You're planning a party…or a dinner out with friends… when all of the sudden a cold sore pops up on your lip.

Cold sores, which are caused by the herpes virus, are nearly impossible to hide, and most medications take days (or longer) to work.

And once you start getting cold sores, they keep coming back—usually at the worst possible time.

But imagine if you could actually reduce the number of cold sores you get, and how long they last.

It's all possible, thanks to a natural amino acid called lysine.

Lysine works by blocking the activity of an acid called arginine, which helps the herpes virus replicate. And the research on lysine and cold sores has been impressive.

In one study out of the Indiana University School of Medicine, men and women who were experiencing recurring herpes infections took lysine three times a day for six months.

They had nearly two and a half fewer outbreaks—and when

the outbreaks did occur, they didn't last as long.

The authors concluded that, "Lysine appears to be an effective agent for reduction of occurrence, severity and healing time" for herpes outbreaks, like cold sores.

Your body can't make lysine, so you must get it from food sources like meat, cheese, eggs and poultry.

And if you want to start supplementing with lysine, it couldn't be easier.

You can buy Nature's Bounty L-lysine supplements at **www.jet.com** for well less than $10 a month. That makes lysine an easy (and affordable) way to start fighting back against those embarrassing cold sores.

Want Better Hearing? Check Your Medicine Cabinet First

Pain is a part of part of life as we get older, whether it's achy knees or occasional headaches.

So like most folks, you might reach for an over-the-counter pain reliever like ibuprofen (the active ingredient in Advil) or acetaminophen (the active ingredient in Tylenol).

While you've likely heard these are bad for your liver, kidney and stomach problems, you may not know there's a new health threat linked to these drugs—one that could alter your quality of life permanently.

This new threat is hearing loss. And research proves that women who take just two ibuprofen or acetaminophen a week could be risking permanent damage to their ears.

For the study, researchers analyzed health data from over 55,000 women and found a significant link between self-reported hearing loss and the prolonged use of ibuprofen and acetaminophen.

After crunching the numbers, they found that women who took these drugs only twice a week over a six-year period raised their risk of developing hearing loss **by almost 10 percent.**

This means simply taking two doses a week could bring you closer to a life of isolation, confusion and limited communication.

These results back a previous study that links over-the-counter painkillers to hearing loss in men. And the bad news only gets worse—the researchers also found that nearly one in six cases of deafness in aging people could be due to painkillers.

While the cause of the link remains unclear, experts believe that these drugs cut the blood supply to your ears, which can cause hearing damage over a long duration.

Fortunately, there's a natural way to cut your pain without reaching for these deafening drugs.

It's called curcumin, and it's the key chemical in the spice turmeric. It can help reduce inflammation and has been a proven pain fighter in several studies.

In one study, folks who suffered from arthritis pain took 200 mg of curcumin daily. At the end the study, they experienced decreased pain and increased mobility. Plus, this dose reduced a series of inflammatory markers, which can up your pain levels.

These types of results aren't shocking when you consider that many studies have shown curcumin to reduce inflammation in several parts of the body.

For other natural pain-relieving secrets, be sure to check out the pain section of this book.

Get Control of Asthma with This Vitamin Fix

If you suffer from asthma (or have a loved one who does) you know you're just one attack away from disaster.

And what does the mainstream medical establishment do to help? They hand you an inhaler and tell you to hope for the best.

Well, that's not good enough—not for you or any asthma sufferer.

Because there's a simple vitamin remedy that can help you cut your number of attacks—and maybe even stay out of the doctor's office or hospital in the process.

Research published in the esteemed Cochrane Library shows that taking oral vitamin D supplements along with regular asthma medication can reduce severe asthma attacks.

Scientists have previously linked low blood levels of vitamin D to increased risk of asthma attacks for both adults and children. More recently, vitamin D has been thought to help reduce upper respiratory infections that may trigger asthma attacks.

For their review, the Cochrane team used seven trials that included 658 adults and 435 children. The participants came from many parts of the world including India, Japan, Poland, Canada and the U.S.

Most recruits suffered from mild to moderate asthma and continued to take their normal medications during the study.

Researchers discovered that taking vitamin D supplements led to a BIG reduction in the risk of severe asthma attacks that required medical attention or a trip to the hospital.

And that's not all. Vitamin D supplementation also reduced the rate of steroid treatments given to folks suffering from severe attacks.

This means taking a daily vitamin D supplement could not only help prevent you from experiencing severe attacks; it may also reduce your need for steroid treatments!

But the best part—the scientists also found that taking these supplements can keep your lungs healthy without any additional side effects.

That's something you can't say about steroids, which can cause weight gain, agitation and water retention and can suppress the immune system.

The best way to get more vitamin D is through sunlight exposure, which helps your body naturally produce it.

However getting outdoor sun exposure during the wintertime (or anytime, for that matter) is not a reliable option for many people, so supplementation is the clear choice for maintaining your vitamin D levels.

You can pick up vitamin D supplements affordably at just about any supermarket or pharmacy, or through an online retailer like **www.iherb.com.**

Delicious Smoothie Fights Even the Worst Jet Lag

You finally hopped on a plane to visit the kids—or to take your dream vacation.

But now jet lag is threatening to ruin everything. Your head is throbbing, you're irritable, and you just can't seem to sleep right.

Jet lag is a common traveling condition that develops when your body's internal clock is out of sync with your destination's local time.

You can try to wait it out and hope it gets better in a couple days. But who wants to waste that kind of time?

Especially when there's a DELICIOUS smoothie that may help you get the upper hand on jet lag symptoms.

The following smoothie is both tasty and healthy for you. The key ingredient is goji berry which is abundant in amino acids and vitamin C that boost your immune system and that your body uses for hundreds of different processes.

Cocoa powder is used for taste and the magnesium contained in it helps to fight fatigue that often comes with jet lag. Almonds give the drink a creamy, milky base.

Directions:

1. Begin by adding 400 ml of water to a blender/smoothie-maker.
2. Add a banana for some extra sweetness and a creamy consistency.
3. Next add cocoa powder (to taste), a handful of goji berries and a glass of almond milk.
4. Blend the mixture together until it becomes smooth.

This wonderfully delicious drink will really boost your energy levels—leaving you in a good mood and ready for anything.

If you get dehydrated when you travel, which is common, there is another healthy drink you can make that will come in handy.

Drinking organic vegetable juice is a great way to rehydrate, detoxify and boost your energy levels in no time at all.

The following juice not only makes you feel better, but it looks, smells and tastes superb.

Directions:

1. Begin by putting four sticks of celery into a juicer. Celery flushes out toxins in the body which can cause tiredness.
2. Next, place two carrots in the juicer. Carrots taste great and help build oxygenated blood.
3. Add half a cucumber. Cucumber is a fantastic detoxifying ingredient.
4. Follow this with a quarter slice of beetroot which gives the juice a sweetness and helps draw out toxins.
5. Next, cut an inch of ginger and place in the mixture.

Ginger aids circulation in the body and masks the taste of the green vegetables.

6. Add a clove of garlic which is another circulation booster that's particularly beneficial for the heart.

7. Last, add some fennel which aids the digestive system in breaking down the juice. It also lends a subtle flavour to the drink.

8. Blend the ingredients together until smooth and serve with ice.

The Medicine Man's Trick for Hot Flash Relief

They call menopause the "change of life." But many women learn the hard way that change isn't easy.

One of the most frustrating symptoms of menopause is those hot flashes that can strike out of the blue, leaving your skin feeling like it's on fire.

Many women have to sleep under a fan—or with the air conditioning turned all the way up—just to get a little bit of relief.

But there's a hot flash secret that Native American medicine men have been turning to for ages, and studies show that it can help get hot flashes under control.

But unless you go to an alternative physician who specializes in natural remedies, odds are you've never been told about it.

Black cohosh, also sometimes known as black snakeroot, is a tall, flowering plant that is a member of the buttercup family. It's found in the eastern, and central United States.

Native American healers have used black cohosh to treat

women's health concerns, such as cramps and hot flashes. Now science is proving that it can help soothe some of the toughest symptoms of menopause.

A study at the University of Illinois at Chicago found that black cohosh seems to reduce hot flashes by targeting the serotonin receptors in the brain. Researchers believe there's a strong connection between serotonin and hot flashes.

The Institute of Complementary Medicine, University Hospital, Zürich, Switzerland, conducted a study of the effects of black cohosh on breast cancer patients, who are very susceptible to hot flashes because of hormone changes from their treatment.

The women who took black cohosh saw a significant improvement in hot flashes, sweating, sleep problems, and anxiety.

And if you're going through menopause, you know that these are four symptoms that can be very hard to shake.

Finally, a study out of Turkey found that black cohosh can relieve hot flashes even better than the antidepressant Prozac, which is commonly prescribed off-label for the condition.

Again, you're not likely to hear about black cohosh at a typical mainstream doctor's office. But it's easy to find online if you know where to look.

You can buy Black Cohosh Meno-Relief at **www.lifeextension.com**. Each tablet comes with 200 mg. of black cohosh.

Take the Sting and Itch Out of Bug Bites in Just *Seconds*!

If you enjoy golfing, working in the garden, or just taking some nature hikes, chances are you've picked up your share of itchy and painful big bites.

They can leave you uncomfortable and scratching your skin raw—and, over time, can even become infected.

But there are easy ways to remove the sting and itch from these bites using items you probably have laying around your house right now.

Here are six worth trying:

#1: Lemon or lime Juice

Lemons and limes are both citrus fruits that can deliver fast relief from insect bites. The soothing effect comes from the citric acid, plus the juice can have an antibacterial effect.

But don't use these remedies if you plan to sit out in the sun, because they can make your skin burn more easily.

#2: Vinegar

The acidic nature of vinegar gives it the ability to soothe the sores left by insects. The best thing to do is wet a tissue or piece of cotton with some vinegar and then place it on the affected area.

The soothing effect should kick in almost immediately, and it is also possible the strong smell will help keep other hungry insects away.

#3: Garlic

Anyone who is familiar with the story of Count Dracula knows that garlic has a reputation for keeping blood suckers away. The good news is it works for predatory insects too because they don't like the smell.

Garlic also contains oils that are natural antibiotics, so rubbing a piece of garlic, or applying some crushed garlic or juice, to the area of the bite is a quick way to make the problem disappear.

#4: Cold tea bags

Don't throw out that old tea bag! Placing a cold, wet tea bag onto the skin will help soothe the irritation and, like garlic, tea is an easily-accessible natural antibiotic.

#5: Essential oils

Many essential oils, including lavender and coconut oil, can be good for banishing the bug bite blues and, thanks to its antibiotic abilities, tea tree oil can be particularly effective.

Many health food stores stock tea tree oil soaps that may create a scent that can keep bugs away.

#6: Toothpaste

Toothpaste may seem like a strange addition to the list, but it's something we always seem to have around.

The majority of toothpastes contain mint or menthol and both compounds have the ability to cool the skin. This can alleviate the pain and irritation of the bite because the "cold" sensation will reach the brain faster than the signals that encourage the need to scratch.

6 Natural Balms Heal Painful Sunburns

We've all had it happen—you spend too much time in the sun or that pricey sunscreen you bought didn't do the job.

Now that bright red, painful sunburn has you looking like a lobster.

But there are some natural balms you can make yourself that can relieve even the most stubborn sunburn pain. And most of them take just a minute or two to prepare.

Sunburn Soother #1: Oatmeal

The beta-glucan in oatmeal acts as a moisturizer and coats the skin to soothe pain and itching.

Cut the end from a pair of old pantyhose at about knee level. Fill the sock with two cups of uncooked rolled oats and tie a tight knot at the top.

Put the oat sachet in the bath and fill the tub with lukewarm water. Squeeze the sock a few times until the bathwater looks cloudy. Soak in your oat bath for 15 to 20 minutes, then allow your skin to air dry.

Sunburn Soother #2: Cucumber

Cucumber has analgesic properties to help reduce pain, and the silica it contains has a cooling effect on the skin.

Take a large cucumber that's been chilled in the fridge, roughly chop it and pulverize it in a blender or food processor. Transfer the puree to a bowl and stir in a heaped tablespoon of corn starch.

Apply the paste to sunburned areas and allow it to dry. Rinse it off with cool water.

Sunburn Soother #3: Peppermint

The menthol in peppermint interacts with cold receptors in the skin for a natural cooling effect. It also helps to reduce the itchiness associated with sunburn.

This remedy takes a little longer to make than the others, but it can be worth it.

Boil a quart of water and add 3 cups of fresh peppermint leaves or 10 peppermint tea bags. Turn off the heat, cover the pot, and allow the leaves to steep for about an hour. Strain out the leaves or remove the teabags and chill the liquid. Soak soft cloths in the infusion and drape them over burned skin.

Sunburn Soother #4: Yogurt

The lactic acid in yogurt stimulates collagen production to promote the growth of new, healthy skin cells.

Use plain, non-sweetened Greek yogurt cold from the refrigerator. Apply a layer to your face, shoulders, and other areas that are badly burned. (You may need a friend to help coat your back.) Leave the yogurt to work for about 20 minutes or until it dries, then rinse it off in the shower. Repeat daily until skin is healed.

Sunburn Soother #5: Aloe vera

Aloe is commonly used to treat minor burns. It reduces pain and inflammation, moisturizes skin and promotes healing.

Cut a long, thick leaf from an aloe vera houseplant (or you can buy a natural gel at the local pharmacy). Use a sharp knife to cut through the side of the leaf and split it lengthwise.

Scrape out the gel with a spoon and transfer it to a container. Gently rub the solution into sunburned skin with your fingers. For extra relief, chill the gel in the freezer before applying it.

Sunburn Soother #6: Vinegar

The acetic acid in vinegar has anti-inflammatory properties to help reduce stinging and itching.

Combine equal portions of vinegar and water in a spray bottle. Mist over burned areas after showering and whenever pain and irritation flare up. There is no need to rinse off the solution. The vinegar smell will quickly fade.

Skip Those *Miserable* Detoxes— And Use This Mouthwash Instead

It seems like every few months or so, some new detox is all the rage. And if you've ever tried a natural detox, you've probably learned that most of them have a nasty secret.

They make you miserable!

Who wants to spend a week drinking cucumber water or kale juice anyway?

But there's an easy way to help your body detox that takes just minutes a day, not weeks.

It's called "oil pulling," and it involves swishing natural oils around in your mouth every day, like a mouthwash. These natural oils can help pull contaminants out of your mouth, which is a main point of entry for lots of toxins.

So how do you oil pull? The most important step is choosing the right oil.

The most popular are sesame, olive and coconut oil and it's important to choose a virgin, cold pressed oil.

Oil pulling should be done before eating, drinking or brushing your teeth, so first thing in the morning is a good time.

Place a teaspoon of the oil in your mouth and begin to swish it back and forth. You only need a teaspoon because the oil will mix with the saliva naturally released in your mouth.

Don't swish too hard, as you have plenty of time and going too fast can make your jaw sore. When you're done, dispose of the oil in the trash bin to avoid clogging the pipes in your sink.

A simple swish for 10–20 minutes (until the oil turns white), done 4–5 times a week, can make a huge difference to your mouth. If you find it difficult at first, start with just a few minutes and work up to longer times.

So why should you oil pull? Here are five great reasons:

#1: Your mouth is the main entrance to your body.

If your body is busy trying to fight mouth bacteria, it has fewer resources to maintain health elsewhere. Keep your mouth healthy, and the rest of your body will be healthier, too.

#2: Your mouth is full of germs.

Depending on what you put in it, you probably have hundreds of types of bacteria growing in the hidden nooks and crannies amongst your teeth and gums.

Although medical professionals say that it's important to maintain regular flossing practices for the tiny places that oil can't reach, oil pulling can help reduce your mouth's bad bacteria.

#3: Mouthwashes and toothpastes are packed with nasty chemicals.

Depending on the brand you buy, you could be exposing your-self to many carcinogenic and unhealthy ingredients. Even if you're good at spitting, you're still going to absorb and swallow many of these chemicals. Oil pulling helps get them out of your mouth.

#4: Oils are loaded with bacteria-fighting ingredients.

Oils such as coconut contain vitamin E and antibacterial properties which can clean and maintain healthy teeth and gums.

#5: You want a brighter, healthier smile

Oil pulling has been shown to both whiten teeth and decrease halitosis (bad breath); so if you're simply interested in how your mouth looks and smells, all the other benefits of oil pulling are just a bonus!

Take a picture of your teeth before you start oil pulling and a month after. You should notice a difference—and hopefully you'll be feeling healthier, too.

Mediterranean Breakthrough Stops Hemorrhoid Pain

Hemorrhoids are the health problem that nobody wants to talk about—but they can make life absolutely miserable.

Veins around your rectum can get swollen and irritated, making going the bathroom nearly impossible and leaving you sitting on pillows all day.

But there's a simple, affordable supplement that you can use to get those swollen, uncomfortable hemorrhoids under control—and we have a group of European butchers to thank for it.

Butcher's broom is an evergreen plant that some people cook and eat like asparagus.

It got its name because Mediterranean butchers used to use its branches to sweep their floors and chopping blocks.

But the more researchers studied this powerful plant, the more they learned that it was good for a lot more than cleaning!

The active chemical in butcher's broom is ruscogen which works in two ways. First, it is a vasoconstrictor, meaning that it tightens veins and improves the quality and tone of capillary walls.

Secondly, ruscogen reduces inflammation which is responsible for the pain and tenderness of hemorrhoids.

By calming inflammation and reducing tissues to their normal size, the ruscogen in butcher's broom helps return your rectal area to normal.

In fact, in one study, 75 percent of doctors rated butcher's broom's effectiveness at treating hemorrhoids as either "good" or "excellent."

Of course, because it's an inexpensive, natural product (and not a pricey drug) don't expect to see any Super Bowl commercials for it.

Butcher's broom is available in powdered root form or as a tincture or tea.

It has a bitter taste as a tea, so it is best to sweeten the tincture or tea with honey, stevia or maple syrup. Prepare the tea by steeping at least one teaspoon of the herb, either loose or in a tea bag, in hot water for 10 to 15 minutes.

You can buy butcher's broom tea at **www.teahaven.com**.

Butcher's broom is also available as a salve or cream for topical application. You can buy Bianca Rosa Butcher's Broom Cream at **www.zooscape.com** (just search or click on the health tab).

This Bible King's Secret REVERSES Vision Loss

It's One of the Most Powerful Sight-Savers Ever Discovered...And It's Finally Headed to America.

They say that your eyesight is first to go—and if you're like a lot of seniors, you've learned that lesson the hard way.

Maybe you've spent years going through thicker and thicker glasses, as the world gets more blurry and less crisp around you.

Maybe you've worried about losing your driver's license... or even your independence.

But, believe it or not, there's a powerful natural substance—one that traces its roots back to the Holy Bible—that can **reverse vision loss** and roll back years on your aging eyes.

For years, the best supply on the planet has been kept from Americans like you, struggling to save their vision.

But all of that is about to change—and you'll never believe why.

PERFECT Vision Thanks to the "King's Spice"

For Paul, total blindness seemed right around the corner.

He'd suffered from glaucoma for more than a decade. He'd had cataract surgery on both eyes, and was due to start receiving painful monthly eye injections.

And that's when he discovered the eye-saving miracle of saffron.

You've probably heard a bit about saffron before. It's a healing spice that comes from a type of crocus flower, and it's been around for nearly 3,000 years.

Believe it or not, we owe its discovery to the same Assyrian King Asenappar that you can read about in the Old Testament's Book of Ezra.

And just like to many herbs connected to the Holy Bible, saffron has turned out to be a certifiable miracle…one that could save your sight or the sight of someone you love.

In fact, Paul experienced the miracle firsthand. In just seven months, he returned for a comprehensive eye exam, and the results were stunning.

His vision had improved dramatically…in fact, his vision field test was PERFECT. And his glaucoma pressure was the lowest it had been in years.

Saffron actually reversed YEARS of vision loss!

And Paul is just one of many people who've had their eyesight dramatically improved by saffron.

In a study out of Italy, patients with early-stage macular degeneration (which can lead to blindness) were given 20 mg of saffron a day or a placebo.

The results were overwhelming: in just three months, the patients who took saffron had improved sensitivity to light and boosted their visual clarity by an impressive 14.3 percent.

Let's put that into some context. That means that someone with 20/40 vision prior to the study improved to

20/30 vision afterwards.

Imagine what that kind of vision improvement could mean for you and your quality of life. No new glasses. No painful eye surgery. Just a safe, natural cure that grows straight from the Earth.

The Healing Power of Saffron

So why is saffron so effective at restoring vision…even vision that may have been fading for years?

Well, as far as your eyes are concerned, it's practically a superfood.

Saffron is loaded with more than 150 active compounds, including carotenoids and antioxidants that have been proven in study after study to improve eye health.

Saffron is like a shield for your aging eyes!

This super spice actually prevents the gradual breakdown of the macula which are light-sensitive cells in the center of the retina.

The degeneration of your macula is one of the leading causes of vision loss as you get older (and can lead to more serious conditions like macular degeneration).

Macular degeneration is actually the leading cause of blindness among seniors.

Saffron is, quite simply, a vision-saving and life-changing natural cure. But for nearly 40 years, most of it has been kept out of the American market.

And it was all thanks to a major international incident you probably remember like it was yesterday.

The Secret Saffron Shortage

None of us will ever forget the Iranian revolution—and the hostage crisis that followed—in the late 1970s.

The United States hit Iran with a major trade embargo, and these sanctions affected a lot more than the oil markets.

What many people don't realize is that Iran controls **90 percent of the world's saffron market**. It's a monopoly.

With so much of the saffron supply cut off to the United States, many in the supplement industry will admit that buying saffron can be a bit of a dicey proposition. You don't always know what you're getting.

Sometimes the saffron is brought into America through dubious third-party suppliers. Often you're buying a heavily diluted mixture with very little saffron (pure saffron, with the supply shortage, can be very pricey), or some sort of synthetic imitation.

"In just 7 months, saffron can restore your vision and significantly reduce glaucoma pressure."

But because of the Iranian nuclear deal you've been reading about for the past year, all that is about to change.

In exchange for promising a scaled back nuclear program, Iran now has trade access to the United States, Canada, and Europe. All of whom are eager to get their hands on the best saffron in the world.

Within the next several months, the best supply of saffron on Earth will begin flowing to United States supplement suppliers. That should bring the quality up and the price down.

And while some Americans will have misgivings about buying anything that originated in Iran, this is one opportunity the Iranians don't want to mess up. They know the market potential is huge, and they're seeing dollar signs.

Our researchers will be following this saffron story closely, and we'll let you know what we find out.

In the meantime, if you want to try saffron to give your aging eyes a boost, make sure you buy from a reputable supplier who is giving you the real stuff.

Saffron Premium (**www.saffronpremium.com**) is a good

place to start, and you'll see its saffron products also marketed for weight loss, where there has been promising research.

You can also check out 100% Pure Saffron Standardized Extract from Gold Source Labs at **www.goldsourcelabs.com**.